Index of Medical Imaging

DEDICATION

For Karen,
Kate and Lucy
who have always supported me in so many ways.

Index of Medical Imaging

Jonathan McConnell

Senior Lecturer, Medical Imaging and Radiation Sciences
Monash University
Melbourne
Australia

WILEY-BLACKWELL

A John Wiley & Sons, Ltd., Publication

Blackwell Publishing was acquired by John Wiley & Sons in February 2007.
Blackwell's publishing program has been merged with Wiley's global Scientific,
Technical and Medical business to form Wiley-Blackwell.

Registered office: John Wiley & Sons, Ltd, The Atrium, Southern Gate,
Chichester, West Sussex, PO19 8SQ, UK

Editorial offices: 9600 Garsington Road, Oxford, OX4 2DQ, UK
The Atrium, Southern Gate, Chichester, West Sussex, PO19
8SQ, UK
2121 State Avenue, Ames, Iowa 50014-8300, USA

For details of our global editorial offices, for customer services and for
information about how to apply for permission to reuse the copyright material
in this book please see our website at www.wiley.com/wiley-blackwell.

Library of Congress Cataloging-in-Publication Data
McConnell, Jonathan.
 Index of medical imaging / Jonathan McConnell.
  p. ; cm.
 Includes bibliographical references and index.
 ISBN 978-1-4051-8544-8 (pbk. : alk. paper) 1. Diagnostic imaging--
Handbooks, manuals, etc. I. Title.
 [DNLM: 1. Diagnostic Imaging--Handbooks. WN 39]
 RC78.7.D53M393 2011
 616.07'54--dc22

                                                              2010052121

A catalogue record for this book is available from the British Library.

This book is published in the following electronic formats: ePDF
9781444340969; Wiley Online Library 9781444340990; ePub 9781444340976;
Mobi 9781444340983

Set in 10/12 pt Palatino by Toppan Best-set Premedia Limited, Hong Kong
Printed and bound in Malaysia by Vivar Printing Sdn Bhd

1   2011

Contents

Index Layout and Acknowledgements

This index is designed to allow easy access to descriptions and discussions of many aspects of medical imaging. It consists of multiple lists, tables and discussions linked to (among others) radiography, computed tomography (CT), magnetic resonance imaging (MRI) and components such as radiological contrast agents, responses to contrast reactions and MRI safety. There is a glossary of terms and definitions plus a list of abbreviations that may be encountered within radiology. Tables are given that suggest the order and type of examination that should be performed as defined by the United Kingdom's Royal College of Radiologists. As a reader all you need to do is find the section you need from the contents list or by thumbing to the position of the item using the thumb tabs on the edge of the pages.

The author, having come from UK practice and having had the opportunity to work in both New Zealand and Australia, hopes the index reflects a wider appreciation of the possible approaches that may be adopted in diagnostic imaging using ionising radiation. Names and terms not seen frequently in one country's practice but described under an alternate label are presented with the intent that this exchange of information will be to the advantage of the patient. Furthermore, in this age of boundary blurring no apology is made for the evident mixture of traditional information that was once the realm of one branch of the profession rather than another.

The index is primarily intended for use by the student or newly qualified radiography practitioner. It may also have value among other professional groups who are also crossing boundaries in their roles or who may be looking for a resource that will support them in their decision making when the computer is unavailable or unable to give an immediate answer in a clinical situation.

Without the help of the following, this index would not have come into being: Jane Carmody, MRI supervisor, Olympic Park Radiology, Melbourne; Geoffrey Dick, CT supervisor, Box Hill Hospital, Melbourne; Peter Kutschera, CT supervisor, Dandenong Hospital, Melbourne.

Chapter 1

Positioning Terminology

The standard anatomical position is assumed, with the individual standing facing the observer with feet turned slightly outwards and hands abducted away from the body and palms flat and visible. In respect to this, several terms can be discussed from this starting position to describe positioning and relations of structures.

Relational terms

Anterior	towards the front of the body; alternative term is ventral
Posterior	towards the back of the body; alternative term is dorsal
Medial	towards the midline of the body
Lateral	away from the midline towards the side of the body
Proximal	towards the origin of the structure
Distal	away from the structure's origin (or further from the body)
Superior	towards the head (cranial or cephalad) or above
Inferior	towards the feet (caudal/caudad) or below
Oblique	from the anatomical position rotation of the body in either direction

Anatomical planes

Sagittal	The mid or median sagittal plane vertically divides the body into two equal (right and left) halves.

Index of Medical Imaging, First Edition. Jonathan McConnell.

Positioning Terminology

Other sagittal planes are subsequently parallel with this.

Coronal   A second vertical plane that can pass through the body to divide it into anterior or posterior sections lying at right angles to the mid-sagittal plane.

Transverse   These are also termed axial planes; the transverse plane divides the body into superior and inferior sections so generating horizontal cross-sections.

Body movements

Understanding body movements is important so that the correct position is adopted for images that may be produced.

Flexion   bending a joint to bring the components closer to each other

Extension   stretching of a joint to separate or elongate joint components relative to each other

Supination   a movement that allows the anterior surface to lie upwards

Pronation   a movement that allows the anterior surface to lie downwards

Adduction   movement of a limb towards the midline (or closer to the body)

Abduction   movement of a limb away from the midline

Inversion   rotation of a joint towards the midline

Eversion   rotation of a joint away from the midline

Internal rotation   rotation towards the centre of the body

External rotation   rotation away from the centre of the body

Decubitus   to lie on a surface of the body and direct a horizontal beam X-ray toward the patient, e.g. dorsal decubitus is to lie on the back with image receptor alongside the patient and effectively a lateral projection is generated by the horizontal ray. Lateral decubitus would have the patient lying on their side.

Chapter 2

Digital Radiography Considerations

Digital radiography, it has been argued, is seen as a massive leap forward in terms of image archiving, manipulation and dose saving. There are, however, a few points that should be remembered when using these systems as the situation is not as simple as it may first appear.

Computed radiography

In computed radiography a photo-stimulable phosphor is the image receptor. X-radiation is captured as a 'shadow' representation of transmission of the beam through the patient, energy amounts being dependent upon what materials the beam passes through, i.e. greater absorption through bone, least through gas-filled structures, and varying according to the thickness of soft tissues elsewhere. The captured energy is released by spraying laser light onto the phosphor; this releases light detectable by a photomultiplier system which amplifies the signal and converts it to a digital data stream. The data stream is then applied to a monitor whereby the data represents grey values on a scale. These are reconstructed in a matrix (pixels) to generate images familiar to the viewer as the radiograph.

Direct digital radiography

Direct digital systems do a similar job but use amorphous silicon or selenium linked to a thin film transistor that has rows and

Index of Medical Imaging, First Edition. Jonathan McConnell.
© 2011 Blackwell Publishing Ltd. Published 2011 by Blackwell Publishing Ltd.

columns of switches equal to the pixel in the image. When the switch is activated the energy stored by the transistor system downloads its information, again as a data stream, though this time a conversion process is not necessary, thus making for a faster response time. These systems are built into equipment as bucky devices or connected to tables and erect stands via cabling or wireless download capabilities so that the receptor can be used in ways similar to (though heavier than) the cassette approach seen in computed radiography.

Patient information

Patient information is applied to each image through the network system termed PACS (Picture Archiving Communication System) which communicates with the Hospital and Radiology Information System (HIS or RIS). The radiographer should ensure an ana-tomical marker is visible in the imaging field, as digital addition of this information afterwards is not best practice.

Exposure and digital radiographic systems

Digital radiographic systems are able to correct for poor exposure factor selection (overexposure by up to 500% and underexposure by about 80%), which at first sounds advantageous. However, this has led to the phenomenon of 'dose creep' whereby imaging staff have gradually increased exposures to avoid image noise generated by underexposure, in the knowledge that overexpo-sure is compensated for by the system. This, over time, has resulted in much higher average exposure factors than those seen in the old film and intensifying screens that gave instant feedback through the analogue image that demonstrated an overly light or dark image. The only way the radiographer can measure the results and relative dose received by the patient is to look at the 'Exposure Index' value delivered by the equipment. This number is a measurement of the energy received by the CR or DR system and corresponds to relative image density. Understand how the system you are working with represents this value, as terms such as 'S value' from Fuji, 'lgM' from Agfa and variations in the posi-tion of a decimal point may lead to confusion; e.g. Kodak gives values between 1600 and 2200 whereas Agfa will display 1.6–2.2 as indications of energy deposited in the system. It is also important to know the speed at which the image was processed. Standard processing would be 100 for extremities, but selection of a faster speed would create the same amount of image blackening for a lower radiation dose. This is advantageous but, if the signal level in the subsystem drops too far, noise is introduced. Furthermore, knowing the speed and exposures can be a useful indication of how to reduce dose while maintaining adequate image quality.

Key elements to keeping dose within acceptable limits and improving image quality include:

- Centralising of the body part to the receptor as images are read from a central point and therefore are electronically adjusted based on this.
- Keeping collimation tight and aligned with cassette edges.
- Using a single cassette per image as this allows shuttering of extraneous screen to improve viewing conditions, better reading of the image data according to selected algorithm and, depending on cassette type, better use of available pixels to enhance spatial resolution.
- Ensuring the correct reconstruction algorithm is applied to the examination. The image may be affected where more than one exposure is added to a single receptor. As a result scatter beyond the collimators causes spurious analysis of the image histogram by the computing system. Take care as each system works slightly differently.

Correct viewing of the image monitor is also crucial to ensuring that a good-quality image is sent to the radiologist's monitor for interpretation. View all images by looking straight at the monitor and not off eye-line, as this can give the impression that all is well with the image when the image quality sent for interpretation is poor. Remember, the radiographer's workstation does not have the same detail functions as the radiologist, so an apparently acceptable image may be grossly unacceptable when viewed elsewhere.

Chapter 3
Plain Radiography Projections

Cross-references in this chapter are to entries in the named projections section in Chapter 4. Projections are suggested singularly on digital cassettes or plates to avoid the issues discussed in Chapter 2.

LOWER LIMB EXAMINATIONS

Foot

ANTEROPOSTERIOR HALLUX (DORSIPLANTAR FIRST OR GREAT TOE)

The patient's shoes, socks and dressings are removed to prevent artefacts. The patient can lie supine on the examination table with a pillow under the head (or sit on the examination table/trolley) with the knee flexed so the foot rests flat on an 18 × 24 cm image receptor. If immobilisation is required, use a large foam pad along the medial border of the leg or flex the other knee to support the affected side.

Use a vertical IR (incident ray) centred to the first metatarsophalangeal joint. Some authors recommend an angle of 10–15° toward the calcaneum to prevent foreshortening of the phalangeal and metatarsal long axes, and correct visualisation of the toe will occur. Ensure collimation to include the neighbouring (second) toe and expose using a 100 cm SID.

LATERAL PROJECTION OF THE TOE

This projection is usually reserved for the hallux as being the structure that bears most weight distally. The affected leg should

Index of Medical Imaging, First Edition. Jonathan McConnell.
© 2011 Blackwell Publishing Ltd. Published 2011 by Blackwell Publishing Ltd.

be rotated medially, facilitated by flexing the affected knee, until the great toe is in a lateral position. To ensure that the toe can be adequately visualised, insert a small foam pad between the adjacent toes and, in the case of the great toe, wrap a small bandage around the smaller toes and extend the bandage around the posterior aspect of the heel. Ask the patient to hold the bandage so that the toes will be pulled inferiorly so that the great toe is separated from its neighbours.

Centre a vertical IR to the metatarsophalangeal joint and collimate to include the digit and metatarsal base.

DORSIPLANTAR OR ANTEROPOSTERIOR PROJECTION OF THE FOREFOOT

Similar to the AP/DP of the hallux, where the patient flexes the knee so the foot can be placed in contact with the 18 × 24 cm image receptor that is positioned transversely, so the forefoot is placed so that it rests on one half. Using a vertical IR, centre to the shaft of the third metatarsal and collimate on four sides to include the whole of the forefoot from toes to the cuneiforms and cuboid.

WEIGHT-BEARING DORSIPLANTAR PROJECTION OF THE FOREFOOT

To show the impact of metatarsus primus varus (precursor to hallux valgus) and the impact of weight on the feet.

The patient stands on the image receptor placed transversely to accommodate both feet at once. Provide a lead rubber full apron as the X-ray tube is brought to a point around the waist while angled 15° towards the patient. The IR is centred between the feet at the mid-shaft point of the first metatarsal and collimated to include the forefeet from mid-foot to toes.

See also: Kandel, Kite, Simmons methods for clubfoot.

OBLIQUE PROJECTION OF THE FOREFOOT

Start with the patient in the AP/DP position and rotate the leg at the hip so that the foot is turned internally and the sole of the foot forms an angle of approximately 30° to the image receptor.

Immobilisation of the patient can be achieved by a number of methods, including the placing of a radiolucent foam immobilisation pad under the raised side of the sole of the foot, or by supporting the medial side of the knee with a larger pad to prevent further internal rotation at the hip.

With a vertical IR, centre to the third metatarsal shaft and collimate to include from toes to the cuneiforms and cuboid at 100 cm SID.

TANGENTIAL PROJECTION OF THE SESAMOIDS

There are two methods.

Patient traction method

Rest the heel on the image receptor and slightly plantarflex/ extend at the ankle. Hook a bandage around the toes of the affected side and ask the patient to pull towards them and downwards to remove the toes from the field of view. Using a vertical IR, centre to the head of the third metatarsal and collimate the beam to include the base of the foot, with the medial and lateral borders both in the field of exposure.

See also: Holly method, Causton method.

Patient prone method

Lie the patient prone on the table with the toes of the foot resting of the image receptor. Flex at the ankle so that an angle of approximately 20° is formed between the vertical and the plantar aspect of the foot. Support the foot accordingly with sandbags and pads, and ensure the long axis of the foot is not rotated relative to the receptor surface. Using a vertical IR, centre to a point at the level of the third metatarsal head. Collimate to include all soft tissue borders.

See also: Lewis method.

ANTEROPOSTERIOR/DORSIPLANTAR PROJECTION OF THE FOOT

Using a 24 × 30 cm image receptor placed in a longitudinal fashion to accommodate the whole foot, place the plantar surface of the foot flat to the receptor and centre the vertical IR to the base of the third metatarsal.

Some centres use a vertical beam, others recommend an angle of 10° towards the ankle to ensure perpendicularity of the central ray to the metatarsal to project a clear joint space. Collimate the beam on four sides to include the whole foot.

(MEDIAL) OBLIQUE PROJECTION OF THE WHOLE FOOT

From the AP/DP position, internally rotate the leg at the hip so the knee of the affected limb turns medially, thus allowing the sole of the foot being radiographed to be raised to form an angle of at least 30° but no more than 45° to the image receptor. Provide immobilisation sponges beneath the foot to prevent movement unsharpness. Use a vertical IR, centre to the third metatarsal shaft and collimate to include the foot and distal end of the tibia and fibula.

See also: Talar neck view and Grashey method for alternative approaches.

LATERAL PROJECTION OF THE FOOT (MEDIOLATERAL)

Turn the patient onto the hip of the affected side, i.e. a lateral recumbent position, and rest the patient's head on a pillow. Flex the leg of the affected side at the knee so the foot turns into a lateral position resting on its lateral border. The other leg is flexed at the knee so the unaffected limb is behind the one being examined.

It may be necessary to raise the knee of the affected side so that the plantar aspect of the affected foot is perpendicular to the image receptor; if so, provide immobilisation. Dorsiflex at the ankle to ensure the ankle joint is also truly lateral. With the foot placed along the long axis of the receptor, use a vertical IR at 100 cm SID centred to a point at the level of the base of the medial or first cuneiform. Collimate the beam to include the distal 2 cm of the tibia.

WEIGHT-BEARING LATERAL PROJECTION OF THE FOOT

Used for the evaluation of pes planus, hallux rigidus and hallux valgus.

With a horizontal IR, place the image receptor on a step stool or custom-built holder, supported vertically with its long axis parallel with the long axis and lateral side of the foot. As the foot is raised into the centre of the image, place wooden blocks in front of the cassette for the patient to stand on.

When standing with the weight being transmitted through the foot of the affected side, the patient may need to support themselves with a handle (preferably secured to the wall). Centre the horizontal IR to the base of the fifth metatarsal (navicular region). Collimate the beam to include the whole of the foot and distal 1–2 cm of the tibia.

See also: Lunge position, Schuss position.

LATERAL PROJECTION OF THE CALCANEUM (OS CALCIS)

As for the mediolateral projection of the foot, but centre the vertical X-ray beam to a point 2 cm inferior to the medial malleolus.

See also: Prayer position.

AXIAL PROJECTION (PLANTODORSAL) OF THE CALCANEUM

The patient is seated on the table with the leg of the affected side extended and the ankle dorsiflexed so that the plantar aspect of the foot is perpendicular to the image receptor. Loop a short bandage around the foot at about the level of the toe bases, so that gentle pressure can be applied to maintain the perpendicularity of the foot relative to the image receptor. This will be uncomfortable for the patient to maintain, especially following injury.

Angle the IR to form an angle of 40° ↑ (i.e. towards the head or, in this case, the ankle joint; ↑indicates up or cranially from IR start position; ↓indicates down or caudally from IR start position) and centre to the base of the third metatarsal – you may need to displace the receptor to capture the elongated image. Use 100 cm SID and employ a kV between 75 and 80 to penetrate the tissue.

See also: Harris and Beam method, Lilienfeld method.

SUBTALAR VIEWS

Although CT has taken over the majority of the imaging of this part of the body, specific areas of the subtalar joints can be evaluated using variation of ↑ angulation (10, 20–30 and 40°) with the medial oblique and just 15° ↑ angulation to show the whole subtalar region with the lateral oblique. A general overview is possible with medial or lateral oblique and 20° ↑ angulation.

Medial oblique
From the AP ankle position, rotate the patient's leg internally so the long axis of the foot forms an angle of 45° to the image receptor. Angle the X-ray tube for each projection as indicated above. Centre to the subtalar region.

Lateral oblique
From the AP ankle position, externally rotate the affected leg so the long axis of the foot forms an angle of 45° to the image receptor. Ensure the ankle joint does not become malrotated as the patient may inadvertently invert the foot. Angle the X-ray tube 15° ↑ from its vertical start point and centre on the talar region, collimating to include the whole of the ankle joint and calcaneum.

See also: Anthonson, Broden I and II, Feist-Mankin, Harris, Harris-Beath, Isherwood methods and Coalition view.

Ankle

ANTEROPOSTERIOR PROJECTION

Patient seated or supine on the examination table (or trolley). Remove clothing, splints, dressings, etc. if possible. Extend the affected limb to rest the heel on a 24 × 30 cm image receptor. Slightly dorsiflex at the ankle so the plantar aspect of the foot is perpendicular to IR. Ensure foot is not inverted at the ankle. Support with radiolucent foam pad if required. Centre a vertical IR between the malleoli and collimate to include at least 10 cm above the joint at 100 cm SID. This image will show superimposition of the lateral malleolus over the lateral joint space.

MORTISE PROJECTION

From AP with 15–20° medial rotation of ankle. Intermalleolar line is parallel to film. Centre vertical IR midway between malleoli. Shows a clear joint space.

LATERAL PROJECTION

Rotate patient to affected side to rest ankle on lateral border. Ensure the foot is coincident with image receptor with no space at toes or heel. Dorsiflex and prevent inversion at the ankle by rotating through the knee and hip. Centre vertical IR on medial malleolus. Occasionally a centring point 3 cm below the malleolus is more successful in demonstrating a clear tibiotalar joint and superimposing the talar domes; alternatively 5°↑ angulation centred on the malleolus is equally successful. Ensure your collimation includes the proximal 2–3 cm of the base of the fifth metatarsal.

OBLIQUE PROJECTIONS

From a mortise position rotate further to enable the ankle joint/foot to form a 45° angle with the IR for a medial oblique. Centre with a vertical IR to the ankle joint to include the distal 10 cm of the tibia and fibula. Conversely, rotate externally 45° to create a lateral oblique projection centred as with the medial description.

STRESS VIEWS

Inversion
To show lateral collateral complex integrity.

Usually performed by the requesting clinician (therefore lead rubber protection should be available) though some centres possess self-stressing devices for patients' use. Begin with the mortise position and ensure collimation light is visible so stressing motion does not lose the area from the radiation field. Allow clinician to stress and make an exposure with a vertical IR on his/her indication.

Eversion
To show deltoid or medial collateral ligament integrity.

As for inversion but allow clinician to evert at the ankle joint.

Anterior draw stress view

To show tibiotalar and talofibular ligament integrity.

Prepare a horizontal ray so that an image receptor lies along the medial border of the foot supported by a pad and sandbag. The patient rests the heel on a wooden block to elevate the whole ankle from the table top. Position as for lateral (i.e. no inversion plus dorsiflexion) and centre to the lateral malleolus. The other leg should be removed from the field for radiation protection. Gently apply a sandbag across the mid-portion of the tibia and allow to remain in place for 1 minute while the patient relaxes. Take an image that includes at least 5 cm of the distal tibia.

Over-rotated lateral projection

To show distal fibula and posterior tibial lip.

From the lateral projection, elevate the heel so the lateral border of the foot is at least parallel with the IR; use a 15° radiolucent pad to support. Patient may have to roll forwards to achieve this position. Centre as for lateral ankle.

Under-rotated lateral projection

To show posterior tibial lip.

From the lateral position rotate the leg so the lateral border of the foot forms a 20° angle with the IR and support with a radiolucent pad. Centre as for lateral ankle.

Tibia and fibula

ANTEROPOSTERIOR PROJECTION

Ideally the whole of the tibia and fibula to include ankle and knee joints should be on the image. This (for most adult patients) will require an increased SID to about 120 cm with a diagonally placed image receptor. Depending on the site of interest it is usually best to ensure that joint position is most true, though having both knee and ankle in AP positions is the ideal. Position to demonstrate as above and centre a vertical IR to fall mid-shaft of the tibia, collimating to include both joints as suggested.

LATERAL PROJECTION

If the patient is able to turn, roll onto side of interest and with a knee flexed to approximately 30° roll the leg onto its lateral side again with the image receptor placed diagonally. Centre to the mid-shaft region with a vertical IR and collimate to include the whole leg.

In trauma situations you may need to take overlapping images of each joint to build a composite image. Lateral projections are attempted lateromedially with a horizontal IR and image receptor placed and supported alongside the medial aspect of the limb.

Knee

ANTEROPOSTERIOR PROJECTION

Place the extended knee joint in the centre of the image receptor. Slightly internally rotate the leg from the hip to place the patella in the centre of the joint. Use a vertical IR and centre to a point 2–3 cm inferior to the patellar apex. Collimate the beam on four sides to include 8 cm of the femur and 2–3 cm below the neck of fibula at 100 cm SID.

LATERAL PROJECTION

From the AP position, turn the patient onto the hip of the affected side and flex the knee to no more than 20°. Place a 15° pad beneath the heel so that the condyles of the femur are brought perpendicular to the film. Angle the IR 5–7° ↑ (towards the femur) and centre to a point 2.5 cm below and posterior to the patellar apex. Collimate the beam on four sides, turning the light beam diaphragm to follow the axis of the tibia such that an appropriate portion of the proximal and distal parts of the joint will be included on the radiograph.

HORIZONTAL RAY LATERAL PROJECTION

Raise the affected leg by placing radiolucent foam pads under the knee joint and also at the ankle if this is required for the patient's comfort. Support an image receptor along the medial border of the knee and rotate the leg internally from the hip until it is in a true AP position. Centre a horizontal IR angled 5–7° to the feet to a point 2.5 cm inferior and posterior to the patellar apex. Collimate to include all the joint at 100 cm SID as for the lateral knee projection.

OBLIQUE PROJECTIONS OF THE KNEE

Medial

To show proximal tibiofibular joint, distal femur, proximal tibia and fibula and the medial half of the patella.

From the AP position internally rotate the leg from the hip, raising the hip if required, should the patient be unable to achieve the rotation naturally, so that the vertical axis of the knee is at 45° to the cassette. Use 100 cm SID and a vertical IR centre to a point 2.5 cm inferior to the patellar apex and collimate to include the same area as for AP knee.

Lateral

Fibular head and neck are superimposed by the tibia, lateral half of the patella is shown clear of the femoral condyles, tibial condyles are projected obliquely so seen in profile.

From the AP knee position, externally rotate the leg so that the knee forms an angle of 45° to the vertical. Centre and collimate the beam as with the medial oblique description.

INTERCONDYLAR NOTCH PROJECTIONS

90°

With the patient seated on the table and prepared for the examination, flex the knee to an angle of 130–140° from full extension. Place an oblong radiolucent foam pad with an image receptor resting on it under the knee, to reduce magnification and provide support for the knee. Angle the X-ray tube so the IR is at 90° to the knee joint and centre to a point 2 cm below the apex of the patella using 100 cm SID.

110°

Exactly the same positioning regime is employed for this projection as for the 90° one, but an angle of 110° relative to the knee joint is employed. An increased exposure may be required depending on the size of the patient's knee as the central ray is more acute. This projection is more useful for the posterior part of the intercondylar notch and may supplement the 90° projection afterwards.

See also: Beclére method, Camp-Coventry method, Frik method, Hughston method.

Patella

POSTEROANTERIOR PROJECTION

Turn the patient onto their front, and extend the legs so that the patient lies flat. Slide the image receptor under the affected knee so that the knee joint and patella are included. With a vertical IR at 100 cm SID, centre to the patella and collimate to include an area similar to the AP knee projection.

WEIGHT-BEARING ANTEROPOSTERIOR PATELLA

Place image receptor in erect stand or bucky. Patient climbs a step and faces horizontal ray X-ray tube (i.e. with their back to the stand). Centre of image receptor is at the level of the knees. IR is between knees. The patient's feet are separated with toes pointing toward the X-ray tube and heels apart to achieve true AP and ensure good balance. Collimate to include both knees on one image, with maximal cover of the leg and thigh achievable by the image receptor depth relative to the patient.

POSTEROANTERIOR PROJECTION WITH FLEXION

See Rosenberg method

POSTEROANTERIOR OBLIQUE PROJECTION

See Kuchendorf method

TANGENTIAL PROJECTION

Look at the following named projections for tangential views of the patella: Brattstrom, Ficat, Hughston, Jaroschy-Hughston, Laurins, Merchants, Settegast, Skyline and Sunrise for variations of approach.

Femur

FULL-LENGTH ANTEROPOSTERIOR PROJECTION

The patient, appropriately prepared for the examination, lies with the affected side extended at the knee so the leg is flat and foot rotated vertically. Place a diagonally oriented (relative to femur) image receptor beneath the thigh so the knee to hip is included when a 120 cm SID is employed. Centre to mid-shaft of femur with vertical IR and collimate to include whole area and give gonad protection where possible. A stationary grid may be applied – remember to check for centring and other cut-off issues.

FULL-LENGTH LATERAL PROJECTION

Rotate 45° to affected side while externally rotating and flexing at the hip so the lateral border of the thigh is in contact with the image receptor. Centre and collimate to the laterally positioned femur as for AP.

SPLIT ANTEROPOSTERIOR AND LATERAL PROJECTION

In trauma or those who cannot move to have the image receptor directly beneath or are too large, two projections that overlap are taken, i.e. knee-up and hip-down. AP projections can be comfortably accommodated in the bucky device. Laterals will have to be obtained using a horizontal IR method. The knee-up approach is an extended version of the horizontal ray lateral knee, to cover more of the femur. The hip-down approach requires the unaffected limb to be lifted and supported on a stirrup or large pad and slightly externally rotated. The image receptor with grid is rested parallel with the neck of femur supported by pads and sandbag or placed in a proprietary holder. The horizontal ray is perpendicular to the neck of femur directed beneath the raised limb and collimated to ensure an overlap between the split images is produced.

For other methods employable in trauma see: Clements Nakayama, Danelius-Miller, Friedman, Kisch, Lorenz methods.

AXIAL SKELETAL EXAMINATIONS

Pelvis

ANTEROPOSTERIOR PROJECTION OF PELVIS

The patient is supine on the table; with the median sagittal plane (MSP) perpendicular, the anterior superior iliac spines (ASIS) are equidistant from the film. The extended legs are positioned with the feet slightly separated so that the toes touch, effectively internally rotating at the hips. Place the patient's hands on the chest and immobilise the ankles using sandbags and foam pads. Ensure the X-ray tube is centred to the bucky tray and place a large image receptor transversely in the tray. Using a vertical IR, centre to a point 2.5 cm above the symphysis pubis in the midline.

The image produced should show the pelvic girdle from iliac crests to include just distal to the lesser trochanters and no asymmetry of structures. Larger patients may require greater than the standard 100 cm SID to be accommodated on the image receptor.

Effect of rotation of the hip joint
With **feet vertical** the true relationship of the femoral head and acetabulum will be better appreciated and more helpful in congenital dislocation of the hip (CDH).

External rotation of the hip will allow visualisation of the lesser trochanter; however, this foreshortens the femoral neck, making fracture detection more difficult.

Internal rotation of the hip joint brings the neck of the femur parallel to the film, allowing better visualisation.

In cases of injury an AP projection of the hip should be taken with uninjured hip in the same degree of rotation as the affected limb. This will allow clear comparison between the two sides for assessment of injury. Any forced movement should be carried out by the requesting clinician if necessary, otherwise the patient should direct how far this movement should occur.

ANTEROPOSTERIOR PROJECTION OF SINGLE HIP

The patient lies supine on the table as for the AP of both hips, with the hips internally rotated. Where possible align a vertical IR to the bucky tray which contains a 24 × 30 cm image receptor. Centre the vertical IR to a point 2.5 cm distal along the perpendicular bisector of a line joining the symphysis pubis and the ASIS of the affected side. (The centring point is directly over the femoral pulse.)

HORIZONTAL BEAM LATERAL PROJECTION OF SINGLE HIP

The patient is supine as for the AP projection of the pelvis. Place a 24 × 30 cm gridded image receptor parallel to the neck of the femur with its proximal border pressed into the soft tissues above the iliac crest. Raise the uninjured limb by flexing at the knee joint to form an angle of 90° and rest in a proprietary leg stirrup attached to the table or a large foam pad.

Centre a horizontal beam IR at a point midway between the greater trochanter and the femoral pulse so that the ray is centred to the grid and at 90° to the film. Collimate to include area of interest at 100 cm SID.

LATERAL OBLIQUE PROJECTION OF SINGLE HIP

The patient lies supine on the table and is rotated through 45° to the affected side (MSP is at 45° to table top) supporting the trunk and unaffected limb with a foam immobilisation pad. Flex the hip and knee joint of the side under examination so that they are in contact with the table top. Ensure the vertical IR is centred to the bucky grid. Use a 24 × 30 cm image receptor in the tray. Centre as for the AP single hip, i.e. at the level of the femoral pulse.

MODIFIED LATERAL (TRAUMA USE) PROJECTION OF SINGLE HIP

The patient is supine with the image receptor positioned as for the horizontal beam lateral. From this position tilt the receptor backwards 25° and support with sandbags and foam pads. Centre the IR to the femoral pulse region at the level of the greater trochanter angled ↓ to be perpendicular to the receptor. Collimate the beam to include the area of interest.

For further suggestions see also: Clements Nakayama, Danelius-Miller, Friedman, Kisch, Lorenz methods.

LATERAL OBLIQUE PROJECTION OF BOTH HIPS – FROG LATERAL (USUALLY CHILDREN)

From the AP pelvis starting position, flex the patient's knees, externally rotate at the hips until the long axes of the femora create an angle of 40–60° with the table top and bring the soles of the feet into contact with each other. Support the legs at the knees with foam immobilising pads and sandbags. Place an appropriately sized image receptor into the bucky tray, centre a vertical bucky aligned IR at a point 2.5 cm proximal to the symphysis pubis and collimate the beam to include both hips/femoral necks. Provide gonad protection if possible, but not at the risk of occluding anatomy which will require another exposure to correct.

OBLIQUE VIEWS OF THE ACETABULUM

See: Judet views

ILIAC OBLIQUE PROJECTION

Side down: shows ilioischial or posterior column and anterior acetabular rim.

OBTURATOR OLIQUE PROJECTION

Side up: shows anterior or iliopubic column and posterior acetabular rim.

ANTEROPOSTERIOR PROJECTION FOR PUBIC BONES

Position the patient as for the AP projection of both hips. Centre the X-ray beam to the bucky but with 20° angulation ↑ for ♂ and 30° ↑ angulation for ♀. Make an exposure at 100 cm SID collimated to include the pubic and ischial rami centred to the lower border of the symphysis pubis.

See also: Taylor method for variations.

PELVIS – INLET VIEW

Position the patient as for the AP both hips, with an image receptor in the bucky. Use an IR angled 40° ↓, already centred to the bucky, to enter the patient at the level of the ASIS in the midline and include the whole of the pelvis.

PELVIS – OUTLET VIEW

Position as for the inlet view (above) but for this projection angle the IR 40° ↑, centring to a point at the inferior border of the symphysis pubis.

See also: Pennal's (Tile's) method that further suggests Bridgeman's method.

Sacro-iliac joints

ANTEROPOSTERIOR PROJECTION OF SACRO-ILIAC JOINT

With the patient positioned as for the AP pelvis, place an image receptor in the bucky tray and centre the IR to the tray with between 10 and 25° ↑ angulation according to the suspected sacral tilt of the patient. Centre the IR at the midline at a point opposite the ASIS and collimate to include both sacro-iliac joints.

See also: Ferguson's method.

POSTEROANTERIOR PROJECTION OF SACRO-ILIAC JOINT

The patient lies prone on the X-ray table so that the MSP is perpendicular to the central longitudinal axis of the couch. Rest the forearms of the patient on the pillow, with the head. Ensure the posterior iliac wings are equidistant from the table and use a bucky-centred IR with 15° ↓ angulation and collimated to the posterior superior iliac spines (PSIS) in the midline. A 24 × 30 cm image receptor should be adequate in size.

POSTERIOR OBLIQUE PROJECTION OF SACRO-ILIAC JOINT

From a supine position rotate the patient 15–20° on to the side opposite the one being examined. Looking down onto the pelvis, the ASIS should lie marginally lateral to the PSIS. Support the patient in this position using radiolucent foam pads. Place an image receptor in the bucky tray and centre the IR that has been angled 15° cranially to the bucky, collimated to include the whole of the sacro-iliac joint, to a point 2.5 cm medial to and 5 cm inferior to the ASIS being examined. A vertical central ray may be used but this will foreshorten the sacro-iliac joint.

STANDING PELVIS – FOR SUBLUXATION OF THE SYMPHYSIS PUBIS

The patient stands with the posterior aspect against the vertical bucky with image receptor in place. Ensure that both ASIS are equidistant from and the MSP is perpendicular to the vertical bucky. With a horizontal X-ray beam centred to the bucky, ensure the symphysis pubis is at the centre of the image receptor so that the IR falls on the symphysis. Collimate the beam to include the hips and expose two radiographs separately with the weight of the body on each leg in turn.

Also termed: Flamingo or Stork methods.

Cervical spine

LATERAL PROJECTION OF CERVICAL SPINE

The patient is erect (seated or standing) with the MSP parallel with and the coronal plane perpendicular to the image receptor (24 × 30 cm). Centre a horizontal IR (perpendicular to the receptor) to a point at C4/5 level which corresponds to a point at the upper end of the thyroid cartilage.

Use an SID of 180 cm. Encourage the patient to relax the shoulders or expose the radiograph on full expiration so that the shoulders are moved downwards.

See also: Grandy method.

ANTEROPOSTERIOR PROJECTION, C3–T2/3

Erect
The patient may remain standing but is turned through 90° so that the posterior aspect of the neck is in contact with an 24 × 30 (or 18 × 24) cm cassette. Ensure the MSP is perpendicular to the image receptor and the shoulders are parallel with it to avoid a rotated

resultant image. Maintain the 180 cm SID and centre with a central X-ray beam angled 12–15° ↑ at the level of the Adam's apple.

This may be achieved with an erect bucky stand though the IR must be aligned with the grid and SID reduced to 100 cm. The exposure factors can remain the same as the reduced SID will effectively counter the impact of the grid on primary radiation.

Supine

The patient lies supine on the table, with the median sagittal plane perpendicular to the table top and coronal plane parallel with it. As with the erect approach, centre IR to the bucky device with 12–15° ↑ angulation. This may be used directly, though some proponents will state that initial centring is to the sternal notch, which is then adjusted by cranially angling the X-ray tube so the central ray passes through the thyroid cartilage. Extend the patient's head and neck so that the occiput and symphysis menti are superimposed. Collimate the beam on four sides to include all the bone and soft tissue structures of the neck to include at least C3 (occasionally a large portion of C2 vertebral body may be visible) and the upper three thoracic vertebrae.

Alternatively a non-grid image receptor may be placed directly under the head and neck – in which case the reduced SID of 100 cm requires a lower exposure factor selection than the bucky method.

OPEN-MOUTH ANTEROPOSTERIOR PROJECTION, C1/2

As with the AP cervical spine, erect and supine options are possible, though many prefer to adopt the supine plus bucky method as this helps patient immobilisation.

The patient extends the neck slightly to enable superimposition of the biting edge of the incisors over the occipital bone. Either a horizontal ray (if the patient is erect) or vertical ray (if the patient is on a table or trolley) are used depending on the technique adopted. Centre the IR which will be perpendicular to the image receptor (bucky and grid where used) and collimate on four sides to include the whole of C1 and C2 which will be neatly framed by the mandible and skull base. It may be necessary to angle the X-ray beam until superimposition is generated.

See also: Fuchs, Judd, Kasabach methods.

WAGGING/MOVING JAW METHOD

Use an open-mouth projection method and select a long exposure time so the patient can open and close the mouth during exposure to reveal the upper cervical spine by blurring the mandible. Particularly helpful in patients treated in a 'halo frame and jacket' for fracture/dislocations of the cervical spine.

Also termed: Otonello method.

OBLIQUE CERVICAL SPINE

Key points

PA obliques (prone): the foraminae nearest to the film are demonstrated
AP obliques (supine): the foraminae furthest from the film are demonstrated

Both oblique projections must be captured to allow for comparison between sides so that neural impingement can be considered. Position the image receptor lengthwise to ensure all the area of interest is included.

Erect posteroanterior
Place image receptor in an erect stand. Ask patient to face stand. Rotate the patient's shoulders so that the coronal plane forms an angle of approximately 50–55° with the receptor so that the shoulder of the side (foramen) to be imaged is closest. Angle of 10–15° ↓ and centre to the middle of the neck at the level of C4 and collimate on four sides.

Erect anteroposterior
The patient's head is in contact with the image receptor with shoulder rotation so that the shoulder (foramen) of interest to be shown will be furthest away from the film. Angle the IR 12–15° ↑ and centre as for the PA projection, remembering to collimate on four sides.

Prone posteroanterior
For this examination the patient lies face down on the X-ray examination table. Centre the IR to the bucky device, tilting the

Plain Radiography Projections

tube ↓ by 12–15°. As with the erect projection, rotate the patient's shoulders to form an angle of 50–55° to the table top. To help maintain this position, bend the knee of the leg furthest from the table top so that it will support the rotated hips. Use the arm and hand of the shoulder turned away from the table top to support the torso. It may be necessary to support the patient with an appropriately sized radiolucent foam pad. Remember that in this position the shoulder that has been raised will be hunched up and so will be projected over the cervical spine. Encourage the patient to move the shoulder down. *Remember that this is uncomfortable for the patient to maintain, especially if forcing the shoulders down.* Centre to C4 and collimate using 100 cm SID.

Supine anteroposterior

The patient is supine on the X-ray examination table. Centre the IR with a ↑ angulation of 12–15° to the image receptor in the bucky tray. Rotate the patient so the shoulder of the side of interest is raised and the torso forms an angle of 50–55° relative to the table top. Support with an appropriately sized radiolucent foam pad and sandbags. Centre the IR to the cervical spine at the level of C4 and collimate using a 100 cm SID.

PILLAR VIEW

Position the patient as for AP cervical spine. Rotate the head 45–50° to the left (repeat for right side) Angle the bucky centred ray 30–40° ↓ and centre the IR just behind the angle of the mandible with the top of the image receptor at the level of the EAM. This is helpful to show the posterior cervical arches, though it has been superseded by CT.

TRAUMA OBLIQUE PROJECTIONS OF CERVICAL SPINE

These projections can be employed to supplement those described above in the acute injury setting.

They allow an oblique projection to be obtained without moving the head of a trauma patient.

45°

With the patient supine on the examination table/trolley, place an image receptor in the trolley tray or directly on the table top so that the edge of the receptor's lateral edge is level with the outside edge of the shoulder. *This may mean the cassette is positioned under the head when the table top method is used. This should only be done under supervision.* Angle the X-ray tube so that it is at 45° to the table top and projects lateromedially, entering the side of the neck at the level of C4.

No grid is necessary but, if one is required for a large patient, ensure the grid lines are running parallel with the direction of the central ray and an SID of 100 cm is used.

60°

To produce a more elongated image of the posterior spinal elements and the vertebral bodies, perform the same projection as above but with a lateromedial angulation of 60°. Although the vertebral bodies will not be projected in good relief, the posterior elements will be shown to advantage so that injury to these regions will be revealed.

HORIZONTAL BEAM LATERAL PROJECTION

The patient lies on the X-ray table or accident trolley. A 24 × 30 cm image receptor, either in a proprietary holding device attached to the table or resting on the trolley or table surface, is placed alongside the neck. Alternatively, where possible, move the trolley alongside the erect cassette stand or bucky to achieve the same outcome. The long edge of the receptor should match the cervical spine long axis.

Centre the horizontally positioned X-ray tube so that the IR passes through C4 and collimate to include the whole of the cervical spine. Use an SID of 180 cm exposure after encouraging the patient to stretch the arms towards the feet so that the shoulders will not be projected over the lower cervical vertebrae. You should have discussed the requirements of the projection prior to exposure so that best co-operation will be ensured.

SWIMMER'S LATERAL PROJECTION, C7–T1

Can be performed with patient erect though more usually the approach is to reveal the lower cervical spine with the patient supine. Patient with hand on head to pull humeral head anterior, other shoulder down and humeral head slightly posterior.

Horizontal IR centred to include whole of cervical and upper three thoracic vertebra. Expose on expiration.

See also: Monda, Pawlow, Swimmer's, Twinings methods.

Thoracic spine

ANTEROPOSTERIOR PROJECTION OF THORACIC SPINE

The patient is supine on the examination table, ideally with the head to the anode end of the X-ray beam (this is to make use of the anode heel effect, if present, to lower the dose of radiation at the upper thoracic region where less exposure is required). Although digital imaging will provide a balanced image, other methods of overcoming this problem include the use of a high kV technique or using wedge filtration on the outside of the light beam diaphragm to correct the beam for satisfactory exposure across the whole of the thoracic spine.

Centre a vertical X-ray beam to the bucky device and collimate to include from C6–7 to the upper lumbar vertebrae. This will give a centring point in the region of the sternal angle in the midline. Ask the patient to hold their breath on inspiration, and expose using 100 cm SID.

LATERAL PROJECTION OF THORACIC SPINE

Lie the patient on the affected side as revealed by clinical history or through evaluation of the AP radiograph. An appreciation of any spinal curvature is necessary so that the fanning effect of the X-ray beam may be employed, so that a correctly exposed radiograph is obtained with obvious clear projection of the intervertebral disc spaces.

Rotate the patient so that the mid-axillary line is perpendicular to the table top. Palpate the spinous processes to assess the degree of angulation that may be necessary to match the slope of the vertebrae. Then tilt the X-ray tube so the beam will match the general direction of tilt of the spine. Centre to a point on the mid-axillary line at the level of the scapula tip or inferior angle (effectively 7–8 cm anterior to the spinous processes) and collimate to include the lower cervical spine to the upper lumbar vertebrae.

Two types of exposure may be made here depending upon departmental preference. A short exposure on arrested inspiration will show the ribs, while a long exposure time as the patient is encouraged to breathe gently will allow the ribs to be blurred out of the image and reveal the spinal structures more clearly.

Lumbar spine

ANTEROPOSTERIOR PROJECTION OF LUMBAR SPINE

Lie the patient supine with the median sagittal plane perpendicular to the table top and with the midline coincident with the central logitudinal axis of the table. (Use of equidistant ASIS as a marker for correct position is often employed. Remember that pelvic rotation as a result of certain pathologies makes this technique less reliable.) A central ray perpendicular to the table top, centred to the bucky device, is employed. To lessen the lordotic exaggeration of the lower lumbar spine some departments ask the patient to bend the knees, which may then be supported underneath by a foam pad, thus allowing better visualisation of the intervertbral disc spaces and the vertebral bodies.

Centre the vertical IR in the midline at a point opposite the level of the lower costal margin which equates to L3. Collimate to include from T11 to at least S3 and laterally to include the sacro-iliac joints – these are often an associated cause for low back pain – as a minimum.

LATERAL PROJECTION OF LUMBAR SPINE

From the AP position, rotate the patient onto the affected side – revealed by clinical indication – or onto the side that will apparently match the fan effect of the X-ray beam as revealed by observation of the AP radiograph. Bend the patient's legs together to aid stability while lying on their side, remembering to ask the patient to rest their hands on the pillow with elbows bent so they are not superimposed over the upper lumbar region. To aid stability in this position it may be necessary to place pads between the knees and any other areas deemed appropriate. Ensure the coronal plane is perpendicular to the table top.

Palpate the spinous processes to ascertain the position attained and if any adjustments need making. Usually, the shape of the shoulders and hips forms a smooth arc which will be matched by the fan of the X-ray beam. There may be a need to alter the direction of the central X-ray beam from vertical to match the slope created by the size of the hips or shoulders. Women require slight ↓ angulation owing to the size of the hips relative to the shoulders – this is reversed in men. An angulation between 3 and 5° is usual.

Centre the vertical IR (when no adjustment is necessary after palpation) 7.5 cm anterior to the spinous process of L3. Collimate to include the area required at 100 cm SID.

OBLIQUE PROJECTION OF LUMBAR SPINE

Reveals the famous 'scotty dog' appearances.

Posterior obliques (supine): display facet joint nearest image receptor (side down)
Anterior obliques (prone or erect with back to the tube): display facet joint furthest from film (side up)

Centre a vertical IR previously aligned with the bucky at the level of L3 along the mid-clavicular line. From the AP projection rotate the supine patient onto the side of interest by raising the opposite side and supporting with a long 45° radiolucent foam pad. To aid stability it may be helpful to ask the patient to reach across with the arm of the raised side to the opposite shoulder. It may be necessary to encourage the patient to bend the knees together and rest towards the side down for comfort. Collimate for the whole lumbar region using 100 cm SID.

ANTEROPOSTERIOR PROJECTION OF
LUMBOSACRAL JOINT

The patient is supine as for lumbar spine. Tilt bucky centred IR 10–25° ↑ ($\male$ = 10° and $\female$ = 20–25° or possibly more). Large angulations may require the image receptor to be moved more cranially in the bucky tray to ensure the image is not projected off the area available for capture.

See also: Ferguson method.

LATERAL PROJECTION OF LUMBOSACRAL JOINT

Maintain the lateral position as described for the full-length lumbar spine. Palpate the PSIS to establish angulation needs of IR. Ensure the coronal plane is perpendicular with the table top. Centre a vertical IR 7.5 cm anterior to the spinous process of L5. This can be confirmed by dropping an imaginary line from the iliac crest approximately 5 cm to meet the line (extended 7.5 cm anteriorly) from the spinous process of L5 or 2.5 cm below the ASIS.

OBLIQUE PROJECTION OF LUMBOSACRAL JOINT

The patient is in the same position as for the oblique lumbar spine. Centre a vertical ray 5 cm medial to the ASIS; if this is not clear, use 10° ↑ angulation of the IR.

VERTEBRAL ARCH POSITION LUMBAR SPINE

Rarely required but useful supplement to CT imaging.

As for the lumbar AP projection except the central X-ray beam must be angled 45° ↓ before centring to the bucky. Centre angled IR in the midline at a point 5 cm above the xiphisternal process and collimate to include the region of interest.

FLEXION AND EXTENSION LATERAL PROJECTION OF LUMBAR SPINE

The projections are performed as a set of examinations to evaluate segmental instability and may be of particular use in those patients that have undergone spinal fusion or are suffering from long-term degenerative changes. There are differences of opinion as to whether the examination should be performed with the patient standing or recumbent. The major deciding factor probably rests with the patient's ability to obtain the positions required.

Standing
With the image receptor in an erect bucky, stand the patient alongside with the lateral aspect of interest nearest the receptor. The horizontal IR is centred to the grid (bucky or other). *Remember* to use a receptor of a size that will accommodate the bending of the patient in either direction.

Standing flexion

Ask the patient to bend forward as far as they can without loss of balance, with the arms and hands away from the sides of the body, possibly rested on the head. Some patients may need some kind of device to hold onto to enable this, which is placed in front of them. Centre to L3 (lower costal margin) and rotate the light beam diaphragm so that it will match the axis of the spinal movement. Expose the radiograph on arrested expiration.

Standing extension

After relaxing the patient from the flexion projection, ensure the bucky has a fresh image receptor in place. Ask the patient to bend as far back as possible without loss of balance, with the hands away from the sides of the body. Collimate the horizontal ray after rotation of the light beam to ensure the axis of the collimation is matched to the spinal axis. Expose on arrested respiration.

Recumbent

To avoid the problems of patient movement and to allow some patients to achieve anything like the kind of position required, it may be necessary to perform the examination with the patient lying on the table. Some practitioners say that the maximum movement can only be obtained by use of this technique over standing. Others state the use of a standing technique gives a better understanding of the effects of load on the spine.

The examination is performed as if obtaining the lateral position with the patient lying on the examination table. From the normal lateral lumbar spine start position, encourage the patient to curl into a tight ball for the flexion view and to arch the back as far as possible for the extension projection. For each exposure, collimation needs to be matched to the spinal axis and performed on arrested expiration.

LATERAL BENDING ANTEROPOSTERIOR LUMBAR SPINE

These projections are intended to indicate any segmental instability in the patient suffering previous trauma or having long-term degenerative disease. They can be performed with the patient standing, or lying on the X-ray examination table. Essentially the same criteria apply to setting up the room as described for the lateral flexion and extension projections, depending on the approach taken.

Centre as for the AP lumbar spine projection but with the collimation set in such a way as to include the area dictated in the AP projection.

Sacrum

ANTEROPOSTERIOR PROJECTION OF SACRUM

With the patient lying supine on the examination table, centre the 15° ↑ angled IR to the bucky device. Centre the IR to a point between the anterior superior iliac spines and the upper border of the symphysis pubis in the midline. Use a 24 × 30 cm image receptor placed transversely in the bucky and expose the radiograph on arrested respiration with factors slightly above those of the AP lumbar spine.

LATERAL PROJECTION OF SACRUM

Rotate the patient to rest on the hip and lateral border of the side of interest. Flex the hips and knees to aid stability. With a vertical IR, previously aligned to the bucky, centre to a point 5 cm anterior to the posterior surface of the sacrum, at the level of the anterior superior iliac spines. Align the light beam field to follow the axis of the sacrum and then collimate.

Coccyx

ANTEROPOSTERIOR PROJECTION OF COCCYX

As for the AP sacrum, lie the patient supine on the table and centre a 10° ↓ angled IR to the bucky, which has a longitudinally placed 18 × 24 cm image receptor in it. Collimate to the area of interest after centring to a point on the midline 5 cm superior to the upper border of the symphysis pubis. Expose at 100 cm SID on arrested respiration.

LATERAL PROJECTION OF COCCYX

Rotate the patient to lie on the side of interest with the knees and hips flexed to aid stability. Centre, with a vertical ray previously aligned with the bucky containing an 18 × 24 cm image receptor, to a point approximately 5 cm superior to the greater trochanter of the raised hip in, effectively, the mid-axillary line. Expose at 100 cm SID using factors similar, surprisingly, to those seen for the lateral lumbar spine.

Spinal curvature radiography

ANTEROPOSTERIOR SCOLIOSIS PROJECTION

Centre a horizontal X-ray to an image receptor placed in an erect bucky. Stand the patient (or position on a stool if they cannot stand) facing the X-ray tube with the back towards the receptor. Centre the beam (and collimate to the spinal region) to the patient ensuring the region of interest will be included, the width of the collimation depending upon the degree of scoliosis present. Avoid any torso rotation if possible, though this may be dictated by the degree of the patient's condition, thus making a nonrotated AP impossible.

Before exposing the radiograph ensure the gonad region is covered. Expose on arrested expiration using a 100 cm SID and a high kV. Although this will reduce contrast by creating more forward scatter, the overall longer contrast scale will allow adequate visualisation of the whole of the spine.

POSTEROANTERIOR PROJECTION

Basically repeat the above but with the patient facing the cassette. As stated this will reduce the radiation dose received by the thyroid and, in women, the breast tissue.

LATERAL SCOLIOSIS SPINE PROJECTION

With a large image receptor placed in an erect bucky, centre the horizontal ray to the grid.

With the convexity of the primary curve towards the film, stand the patient so they are lateral to the beam and rest the hands on the head. To ensure there is an even exposure, a compensating wedge filter could be used with the thin end towards the lumbar spine (digital capability now makes this less necessary).

Centre the X-ray beam to the midpoint of the spine (T10 region) and collimate to include the whole of the vertebrae as outlined. Expose on arrested expiration at 100 cm SID with factors in the region of 90–100 kV.

RIGHT AND LEFT BENDING PROJECTIONS

Repeat the AP (or PA) technique but make separate exposures when the patient has bent maximally to the left or right. These projections will highlight segmental stability from a lateral point of view.

UPPER LIMB EXAMINATIONS

Hand and wrist

POSTEROANTERIOR PROJECTION OF HAND

Place the patient's hand palm down, with fingers slightly separated, on the image receptor. Ensure the hand is not cupped in any way and the wrist is parallel with the receptor. Centre a vertical IR to the head of the third metacarpal and collimate to include the digits and wrist.

POSTEROANTERIOR OBLIQUE (DORSIPALMAR OBLIQUE) PROJECTION

From the PA position rotate the hand towards the lateral position (externally) until the palm of the hand forms a 45° angle to the image receptor. Centre a vertical IR to the head of the fifth metacarpal and collimate as for PA.

LATERAL PROJECTION

The hand is rotated onto the ulnar aspect of the fifth metacarpal with fingers outstretched. The thumb is supported on a radiolucent foam pad. The carpus and metacarpals will be superimposed, which is correct for fracture angulation evaluation and foreign body detection. Centre a vertical IR over the head of the second metacarpal and collimate to include the thumb and dorsal aspect of the digits and wrist.

STEEP EXTERNAL OBLIQUE

Rotate from the lateral position approximately 20° posteriorly (towards the dorsum of the hand) so the thenar eminence of the thumb is no longer superimposed over the head of the fifth metacarpal. Centre the vertical IR on the head of the fifth metacarpal and collimate to include the whole of the fifth digit and metacarpal. This view aids evaluation in fractures where superimposition of other structures is problematic.

Fingers

POSTEROANTERIOR PROJECTION

As for PA hand except centre the vertical IR over the head of the metacarpal of the digit of interest. Collimate to include the metacarpal and ensure the adjacent fingers are at least partially in the radiation field to aid identification of the specific digit.

LATERAL PROJECTION

Index and middle fingers

Internally rotate the hand via the shoulder so the radial border of the index finger rests on the image receptor. To show the index finger in lateral profile extend the digit and bunch the remaining fingers together to avoid superimposition. Centre a vertical ray on the proximal phalanx, ensuring that no rotation or horizontal angulation (relative to the image receptor) of the finger is evident. For the middle finger, repeat the process except extend the digit of interest and insert a radiolucent pad between the extended finger and those bunched away, to ensure true finger extension and minimal opportunity for movement unsharpness. Again check for angulation so that interphalangeal joint spaces will be clear.

Ring and little finger

The process is very similar except the hand is externally rotated to rest on the ulnar border of the fifth metacarpal. The little finger is extended in this case and the remaining fingers bunched. Centre as described for the index finger. The ring finger should be separated in a fashion as described for the middle finger, again remembering to be vigilant for evidence of rotation or angulation.

Fan view

Some practitioners will support the idea of fanning all fingers to obtain laterals of each finger. This should be avoided as rarely is this view fully successful with all joint spaces being clear and bones correctly displayed.

Thumb

ANTEROPOSTERIOR PROJECTION

The patient is seated or kneeling at the table end. The arm is first extended along the table with palm down and elbow straight. Internally rotate from the shoulder until the posterior aspect of the thumb may rest on the image receptor. Extend the fingers to avoid superimposition of digits or the thenar eminence of the fifth metacarpal. Centre a vertical IR to the metacarpophalangeal joint (MCPJ) and collimate to include the phalanges and the carpal bones.

LATERAL PROJECTION

From the PA hand position, internally rotate the hand by lifting the fifth metacarpal until the thumb forms a lateral profile. Support at the fifth metacarpal with a radiolucent pad and centre to the MCPJ, collimating as for the AP projection.

POSTEROANTERIOR PROJECTION

If the patient cannot achieve the position described for the AP thumb (e.g. trauma or movement disability) rotate the hand from the PA to lateral position with the thumb extended and supported by a radiolucent foam pad. Centre the IR to the first MCPJ – some texts indicate an increased SID to counter any magnification effects.

See also: Lewis method, Long-Rafert method, Robert's method.

Metacarpals

It is unusual to request metacarpals as a separate examination; more usually these are a supplementary projection to the hand.

Check the following named approaches: Ball catcher or Norgaard method – AP oblique hand, Betts – first carpometacarpal joint, Brewerton – metacarpal heads, Burman – first carpometacarpal joint, Carpal boss – carpometacarpal joint.

Wrist joint and carpal bones

Often as a first attendance (especially post trauma) the wrist is the standard examination that evaluates the carpal bones as well. As such the area of interest would be from the metacarpal bases to include 6–8 cm of the radius and ulna.

POSTEROANTERIOR (DORSIPALMAR) PROJECTION

The patient's forearm is pronated onto the image receptor ensuring the wrist is fully in contact. This may require the fingers to be slightly flexed or supported on the ulnar side by a radiolucent pad to prevent rotation. Centre a vertical IR midway between the radial and ulnar styloid processes. Collimate as suggested above.

LATERAL PROJECTION

From PA externally rotate to rest the hand (through the elbow and shoulder) on the ulnar border of the fifth metacarpal. Rotate 10° past vertical to superimpose the radius and ulna. Note – rotating merely by turning the hand will not clarify problems with ulnar variance and reveal true superimposition. Centre the vertical IR to the radial styloid process and collimate to include the area as suggested above.

POSTEROANTERIOR OBLIQUE PROJECTION

From the PA position rotate towards the lateral so the palm forms an angle of 45° to the image receptor. Support with a pad under the thumb and centre the vertical IR to the ulnar styloid process. This projection may be collimated as for full wrist or to encompass purely the carpal bones.

ANTEROPOSTERIOR OBLIQUE PROJECTION

A nonstandard projection today, 'Stecher's view' will frequently be taken as a four-view carpal evaluation series, especially for possible scaphoid fracture. However, from the lateral position, rotate posteriorly until the dorsum of the wrist is angled 45° to the image receptor. Centre the vertical IR to the ulnar styloid and collimate appropriately for the clinical question. Both the obliques may be taken in ulnar flexion (deviation) when evaluating for scaphoid fracture.

See also: Burman – first carpometacarpal joint, Carpal boss – carpometacarpal joint, Carpal bridge – tangential carpus, Carpal canal projection, Daffner, Emmerling and Buterbaugh – scaphoid and capitate, Gaynor-Hart – carpal tunnel, Lentino – carpal bridge, Rafert-Long – scaphoid, Stecher – scaphoid, Templeton and Zim – carpal tunnel, Ziter method – scaphoid.

Stress projections of the carpus may also be performed by simply repeating the PA and lateral (and possibly the PA oblique) by obtaining all views with clenched and unclenched fist or radial and ulnar flexion (deviation).

Forearm

ANTEROPOSTERIOR PROJECTION

The patient is seated with the forearm extended and posterior aspect and dorsum of the hand resting on the image receptor such that a true AP elbow position is achieved. Centre a vertical IR to the mid-shaft of the radius and ulna and collimate to include both wrist and elbow in the image.

LATERAL PROJECTION

Ensure the upper arm is on the same plane as the forearm, which is resting in a lateral position (wrist and elbow) on the image receptor. Centre a vertical IR to the mid-shaft region and collimate to include both joints.

TRAUMA POSITION

In a trauma situation it is unlikely that the true AP and lateral positions will be achievable for the patient. Instead a composite pair of images can be obtained with the elbow positioned laterally and wrist PA and conversely with the wrist truly lateral and an AP elbow. Make use of any ability to manipulate the height of the table as this will ensure the patient can achieve and hold these positions.

Alternatively, if the first position indicated above can be obtained the use of a horizontal ray and image receptor along the radial or ulnar border to achieve the orthogonal composite view may be feasible without further movement of the patient.

Elbow

ANTEROPOSTERIOR PROJECTION

Extend the arm at the elbow and rest it on the image receptor, ensuring the whole arm rests on a plane with the shoulder. Centre a vertical IR to a point 2.5 cm inferior to the humeral condyles and collimate to include 6–8 cm either side of the skin crease of the joint.

LATERAL PROJECTION

The elbow and wrist are positioned in the true lateral projection if this can be achieved (see comment under forearm). Ensure the elbow and shoulder are on the same plane and the wrist is not higher or lower than the elbow (i.e. rotated through the long axis). Centre to the lateral epicondyle with a vertical IR and collimate as suggested for the AP.

FLEXED ANTEROPOSTERIOR PROJECTION

When extreme flexion is the only position the patient will adopt, rest the posterior surface of the humerus on the image receptor. The patient will support the forearm with the other hand. Centre the IR with 10–15° ↑ to the shoulder and collimate to include the whole joint.

See also: Jones – flexion elbow.

PARTIALLY FLEXED ANTEROPOSTERIOR PROJECTION

Equal angles
If the patient is unable to fully extend the elbow, obtain an AP position with equal angulation of the forearm and humerus

relative to the image receptor plane (a pad to support the wrist may be helpful). Centre at the elbow crease and collimate to include 6–8 cm either side of the skin fold. *Note* this view will not produce a clear joint space and so cannot be used to evaluate articular surface damage.

Flexed forearm and humerus favoured projections
Rather than the equal angles approach, obtain a true distal humeral AP as discussed for the full elbow AP. Support the wrist of the flexed elbow and centre on the humeral condyles. This view will show the humeral articular surfaces. Repeat with the forearm resting fully on the image receptor and centre the vertical IR 1 cm below the elbow skin crease. This view will reveal the radius and ulna articulations.

ANTEROPOSTERIOR PROJECTION OF HEAD OF RADIUS

Slightly flex the patient's elbow, resting on the point of the joint to rotate externally approximately 30° so the head of the radius is tangential to a vertical IR centred to the skin crease.

See also: Capitellum projection (Berquist method), Coyle trauma methods, Tomas and Proubasta – radial head, Tuberosity view – elbow.

ULNAR GROOVE (SUPERO-INFERIOR) PROJECTION

Seat the patient with their back to the table. Flex the elbow and extend at the shoulder to bring the elbow back to rest on the image receptor, i.e. resting on the elbow. The humerus should form an angle of 25–30° to the vertical. Centre with a vertical IR to the ulnar groove found slightly lateral to the medial epicondyle.

See also: Laquerriere and Pierquin method, Pierquin method, Veihwëger method.

Humerus

ANTEROPOSTERIOR PROJECTION

If size image receptor permits, both the shoulder and elbow should be included on the final radiograph. The patient may be erect or supine and rotated slightly (15–25°) towards the affected side so a true AP (anatomical man) position can be adopted. Centre to the mid-shaft of humerus and collimate to include both joints.

LATERAL PROJECTION

Erect position enables easier manipulation of the patient; this could be standing or seated. The patient faces the image receptor and bends the elbow (trauma situations would usually see the patient supporting the forearm) to bring the forearm across the abdomen. Rotation at the shoulder achieves a lateral projection; slight separation of the elbow from the trunk is recommended to enable a clear projection to be achieved; this also puts the patient into a position where a slight bending forward ensures good object-to-receptor contact. Centre to the mid-shaft of humerus using a horizontal IR.

TRANSTHORACIC LATERAL PROJECTION

Rarely performed now due to radiation exposure concerns. However, a horizontal ray can be projected through the thorax after the unaffected arm is lifted from the field. Patient is alongside the receptor which may be in an erect stand or bucky device. Position the grid so it matches the centre of the humerus; thus centring to the bucky ensures no grid cut-off and inclusion of the whole area on the radiograph.

Shoulder girdle

ANTEROPOSTERIOR PROJECTION

To show the glenohumeral joint (GHJ) clearly, the patient should be rotated approximately 45° towards the affected side. The arm is positioned as for a true AP and horizontal IR centred at the coracoid process. Collimate to include the whole shoulder. This projection will show the clavicle as foreshortened; to see the clavicle, position the patient with 10–15° of rotation to the affected side.

LATERAL PROJECTION OF HUMERAL HEAD

Adopt a position as for the lateral humerus by adducting the arm across the chest and support with the unaffected hand but centring the horizontal IR to the GHJ with the patient in an AP position. DO NOT attempt this if there is injury; a horizontal ray lateral of the humeral head may be used if radiation dose is acceptable.

SUPERO-INFERIOR PROJECTION

Place an 18×24 cm image receptor beneath the axilla of the patient who has abducted the humerus across the table while seated alongside. This is possible if the elevation options for the examination table are employed. The patient will have to tilt the head away from the affected side to avoid artefact generation. Centre the vertical IR to the GHJ. Depending on the distance from the receptor a compensatory increase in SID (and exposure) may be used to counter magnification.

INFEROSUPERIOR PROJECTION

This approach is particularly helpful for the trauma situation. The patient is supine and receptor supported by a pad and sandbag to be parallel with the superior surface of the shoulder. The arm is abducted away for the shoulder (ideally 90°) though in trauma this is unlikely. Support the abducted arm and with a horizontal IR directed towards the GHJ and centre to the axilla. Where the patient is unable to abduct the arm significantly, a larger SID will enable the X-ray tube to be positioned alongside the patient to obtain a shallower angled/tangential line of IR to produce a radiograph of the ideal position discussed earlier.

Both the above are good projections for the acromion and cora-coid processes.

Multiple specialist views have been developed for shoulder evaluation. The following named views should be adopted for the given clinical uses:

Adams – prone, Blackett-Healy – prone tangential, Didiee view – prone, Fisk – bicipital groove, Garth – trauma dislocation, Grashy – true AP, Hermodsson's – internal rotation and tangential, Hill-Sachs defect, Johner – supine tangential, Lawrence – proximal humerus, transthoracic, Miller – query dislocation, Neer – outlet, Oppenheim – cephaloscapular projection, Outlet view – for humeral impingement, Stryker – posterior humeral head, Supraspinatus outlet view – acromion, Wallace-Hellier – AP, West Point view – glenoid rim, prone, Y view – axial shoulder or lateral scapula.

Scapula

ANTEROPOSTERIOR PROJECTION

Rotate the erect or supine patient externally so the scapula is parallel with the image receptor. Centre the IR to be perpendicular to the receptor and over the humeral head to throw the thoracic cage away from the scapula, thus rending clearer visualisation.

LATERAL PROJECTION

Prone or erect
The patient faces the image receptor (in a bucky device or grid that has been applied) and rotated 30° towards the affected side. Abduct the arm across the body to rest the hand on or in front of the opposite shoulder. Palpate the scapula to ascertain if it is perpendicular to the image receptor. Use a horizontal IR centred to the upper one-third medial border and collimate to include the whole scapula blade, spine, acromion and coracoid processes.

Supine
Encourage the patient to abduct the affected arm across to the opposite shoulder. Rotate the affected side away from the table until the palpated scapula is perpendicular to the image receptor. Centre the vertical IR over the glenoid area and collimate as suggested for the prone/erect approach.

See also: Laquerriere and Pierquin – supine scapula, Y view – axial shoulder or lateral scapula.

Clavicle

ANTEROPOSTERIOR PROJECTION

With an erect or supine patient adopt a position as for the scapula. Collimate the IR to include the whole of the clavicle, though inclusion of all the scapula blade is not necessary.

See also: Alexander method, Alexander stress method, Pearson method, Zanca's method – acromioclavicular joint.

POSTEROANTERIOR PROJECTION

The patient is either prone or erect facing an image receptor. A horizontal IR is directed towards the mid-clavicle after the patient has been rotated towards the receptor 10–15° so the clavicle is parallel with the stand or bucky.

See also: Quesada method – clavicle prone.

LORDOTIC – AXIAL PROJECTION

Erect patient
The erect patient (seated or standing) is asked to lean back 25–30° towards the image receptor held in a bucky or proprietary stand. A horizontal IR is directed to the midpoint of the clavicle and collimated to include the area indicated for the AP projection.

Angled tube
If the patient is unable to adopt a lordotic position, encourage to rest against the image receptor, then angle the IR 30° ↑ and centre on the midpoint of the clavicle.

A combination of angulation and/or the patient adopting lordosis posture can be employed to achieve the same outcomes.

INFEROSUPERIOR PROJECTION

This projection is useful for showing fragment displacement post fracture. The patient is supine and the image receptor supported along the upper border of the shoulder. The IR forms an angle of 45° to the receptor and is centred mid-clavicle, ensuring the whole bone is included in the collimation. This will require the receptor to be tightly pressed against the neck of the patient and may require some tilting of the head away.

Acromioclavicular joint

ANTEROPOSTERIOR +/– STRESS VIEWS

Position as for AP shoulder and centre the horizontal IR just above the humeral head, with the beam collimated to include the

ACJ. Both sides should be examined to compare and are then repeated with a sandbag in each hand to pull against the relaxed shoulder. Resisting the sandbag's pull undermines the stress, stopping evaluation of potentially disrupted ligaments.

See also: Alexander – acromioclavicular joint, Alexander stress method – acromioclavicular joint, Pearson – acromioclavicular joint, Zanca's view – acromioclavicular joint.

Sternoclavicular joint

ANTEROPOSTERIOR PROJECTION

The patient is erect with both arms hanging in relaxed fashion by the sides. Centre to the manubrium sterni with a horizontal IR and collimated to show both SCJs on the 18 × 24 cm radiograph.

POSTEROANTERIOR OBLIQUE PROJECTION

The patient is erect or prone, i.e. in PA position. Rotate 45° to bring the side of interest closer to the image receptor and centre to this SCJ using an IR perpendicular to the stand or bucky. Repeat for the opposite side.

EXAMINATION OF THORAX AND CONTENTS

Sternum

POSTEROANTERIOR OBLIQUE PROJECTION

From a true PA position, rotate to each side 30° and centre with an IR perpendicular to the image receptor to the mid-sternal area. Collimate to include the whole sternum.

POSTEROANTERIOR PROJECTION

This approach cannot be taken across the grid lines of the bucky mechanism though it is possible if the IR runs parallel with the axis of the grid lines. Position the patient in a true PA and then angle the IR 30° to the midline. A long exposure time may be used to blur the ribs as the image is taken on gentle respiration.

LATERAL PROJECTION

The patient is erect and in the true lateral position relative to the image receptor. Clasp the hands behind the back and draw the shoulder back as far as the patient will achieve. Centre to the mid-sternal region with an SID similar to the chest due to the large object-to-receptor distance and possible magnification problems. Expose on arrested respiration.

For the trauma situation the patient may be supine; in this instance a horizontal cross-table IR is used with the image receptor held in an erect bucky or stand. The patient is encouraged to raise the arms away from the irradiated area to reveal a true lateral radiograph of the lateral sternum.

Ribs

From a radiographic perspective ribs are divided into upper and lower to account for anatomical shape, overlying structures and likely approaches to exposure technique. It is arguable that the rib image has little value as management does not change significantly in most cases unless a pneumothorax or flail segment is present, in which case differing treatment approaches will have been likely from the outset.

UPPER RIBS

Anteroposterior projection
Patient is in true AP position against a large image receptor. Centre the IR to be perpendicular with the receptor at the level of the sternal angle. Collimate to include the maximum number of ribs possible in a single exposure on arrested inspiration.

Posteroanterior projection
Start with a true PA position and rotate the affected side towards the receptor. Collimate to maximally cover the ribs and expose on arrested inspiration.

Posterior oblique projection
This view allows the side of interest to be in contact with the image receptor. Rotate the patient's posterior aspect 45° to the affected side and place the arm of that side on the head. Centre

to the receptor and collimate to cover the maximum number of ribs in the area.

LOWER RIBS

Anteroposterior projection
A large image receptor placed transversely will enable both sides to be obtained in a single exposure. Angle the IR 10° ↑ to maximise the subdiaphragmatic ribs contained on the single exposure and centre at the level of the lower costal margin in the midline (if a single side is imaged, centre to the mid-clavicular line of that side). Expose on full expiration to maximise the overall abdominal area covered by those factors.

Posterior oblique projection
Rotate to the affected side 45° from the AP position. Angle the IR 10° ↑ to reduce the collimation size over the rest of the abdominal contents. Centre the IR to the midline, which has now rotated into the field, and expose on arrested expiration.

See also: Williams method – costovertebral and costotransverse joints.

Chest

Unless stated otherwise, all views are obtained at 180 cm SID.

POSTEROANTERIOR PROJECTION

The patient is erect, facing the image receptor which is positioned to include the root of the neck to the pulmonary bases. Place the backs of the hands on the hips and rotate arms and shoulders forwards to project the scapulae from the lung fields, ensuring the MSP remains perpendicular to the receptor. Centre with a horizontal IR to the fifth thoracic vertebra. Some practitioners advise that the beam be angled 5° ↓ from this centring point to enable collimation that covers the chest but will be below eye level and minimal towards the thyroid. Expose on arrested inspiration; for pneumothorax detection a second image may be obtained on expiration to attempt to expand the size or change the position of the lesion and make it visible, though some references suggest this is of minimal value.

LATERAL PROJECTION

The patient is erect with the side of interest towards the image receptor. Place the hands on the head and bring the elbows close together in front and as high as possible. Some equipment offers a handle for patients to use in this way but the same principles apply. Centre with a horizontal IR through the axilla at T5 and collimate to include the whole chest.

ANTERIOR OBLIQUE PROJECTIONS

Right (right anterior oblique)
From a PA erect position place the left hand on the head and rotate the body so the right side moves towards the image receptor to form an angle of 60° with it. Centre with a horizontal IR at T5 and collimate to include the whole chest.

Left (left anterior oblique)
As for the right but rotate the left side toward the receptor to form an angle of 70° and centre as above.

APICAL VIEW (ANTEROPOSTERIOR)

From an AP position approximately 30 cm in front of the image receptor, lean the patient back to rest on the image plate. Centre a horizontal IR to the midline at a point 7.5 cm below the horizontal plane of the clavicles. Slightly bend the elbows and rotate the arms internally from the shoulders to move the scapulae away from the field. Expose on arrested inspiration. Alternatively, if the patient is unable to bend this way, angle the IR 25° ↑ and centre to the apices (see lordotic clavicle).

LORDOTIC VIEW

This projection aids detection of right middle lobe collapse or right-sided interlobular pleurisy. From the PA position ask the patient to bend backwards 30° by holding the erect stand as support, centre the horizontal IR to T5 and expose the whole chest on inspiration at 100 cm SID.

ANTEROPOSTERIOR PROJECTION

This projection is employed where patients cannot sit or stand safely. The image receptor is placed behind the patient, who is either in a wheelchair and hence relatively erect, or supported on a trolley by a large 45° foam pad rested against an angulated trolley back. A lordotic position is easy to adopt here so take care to ensure the IR is perpendicular to the image receptor. Collimate to include the whole chest, centring to the sternal angle.

SUPINE VIEW

The least favourable position for cardiac evaluation. However, this may be the only option for some patient presentations. Place the image receptor either directly under the patient or, more probably, in a trolley tray, which causes magnification problems. Use the largest distance possible and consider lowering the trolley or bed height to achieve this. Lordosis may be problematic, especially in younger patients where the head tips backwards. In these cases provide a cushion or sponge or, if very young, consider angling the image receptor to counteract the problem. Collimate to include all of the chest and expose on inspiration.

LATERAL DECUBITUS PROJECTION

Rarely used in the chest today as CT is able to reveal more information about fluid compared with plain images.

The image receptor is held in an erect stand or bucky and horizontal IR centred to it. The patient turns onto the side, as described above, so the beam could travel AP or PA through the patient and the IR is centred to include all the chest when collimated. The image is preferably taken on arrested inspiration. Ensure the patient is elevated from the table or trolley surface so a full evaluation of any fluid levels can be made.

Thoracic inlet

ANTEROPOSTERIOR PROJECTION

The patient is supine or erect in true AP position, with chin raised. Centre a perpendicular IR to the sternal notch and collimate to tracheal and mediastinal areas. This projection may be supplemented with a soft-tissue AP cervical spine, and is usually performed on arrested inspiration at 100 cm SID. It is supplemented with a Valsalva manoeuvre image to show the impact of air under pressure on the trachea and laryngeal regions.

LATERAL PROJECTION

The patient is erect, in the true lateral position with the hands clasped behind the back. Centre a bucky-centred horizontal IR to the sternal notch, then ask the patient to push the shoulders further back, so the tracheal space in the mediastinum is revealed in front of the shoulders on the image receptor. Expose on arrested inspiration; a repeated image with a Valsalva manoeuvre may be required. A lateral soft-tissue cervical spine usually accompanies this view to reveal the whole trachea, nasopharynx and oropharynx.

EXAMINATION OF ABDOMEN AND CONTENTS

Abdomen

ANTEROPOSTERIOR PROJECTION (SUPINE OR ERECT)

The patient is supine with the lower border of the image receptor at the level of the symphysis pubis. Centre with an IR perpendicular to the midline to the middle of the receptor. Collimate to include abdominal contents that will fit the receptor size, and expose on inspiration.

For erect images it is ideal if the patient can stand against a bucky device. However, arguments persist about the value of the examination in light of CT, the dubious nature of obstructive appearances on plain images and the fact that an erect chest will show perforation effects far more clearly.

ANTEROPOSTERIOR PROJECTION OF RENAL AREA/DIAPHRAGM

This image is taken to show the renal zone but with a larger image receptor placed transversely it may be used to create a composite abdominal examination in larger patients. Centre the

IR to the midline at a point midway between the xiphisternum and lower costal margin. Collimate to include either the renal area or wider if wishing to demonstrate the diaphragmatic zone.

DECUBITUS PROJECTIONS

In describing the decubitus projection (performed where an erect image is required but the patient is unable to be erect), decubitus means 'laid down' to which are added 'lateral + side' to say the patient lies on a given body surface. A right lateral decubitus indicates the patient is lying on the right side so the left flank is observed for free gas and right for fluid collections. The dorsal decubitus indicates the patient is supine and the anterior abdominal wall is the dependent area to observe for free gas.

Lateral decubitus projection

The image receptor is held in an erect stand or bucky and horizontal IR centred to it. The patient turns onto the side as described above so the beam could travel AP or PA through the patient and the IR is centred to include maximal amounts of abdomen when collimated. The image is preferably taken on arrested inspiration.

Dorsal decubitus projection

The patient is on their back, ideally elevated clear of the table or trolley surface by a radiolucent mattress. A horizontal IR centred to the receptor in the bucky or stand is centred to the midpoint of the abdomen. Collimation is performed to maximise cover; however, bear in mind that burnout could occur at the soft tissue/air interface if inappropriate exposure factors are selected.

Hepato-biliary

GALLBLADDER

Posteroanterior projection

The patient is prone (or erect) facing the image receptor in the bucky. For prone, rest the left arm by the side and right hand on a pillow at the head to create moderate rotation away from the receptor. Centre a vertical IR 10 cm right of the spine at the level of the lower costal margin.

Anteroposterior (posterior oblique) projection
The patient is supine on the table, with IR centred to the image receptor in the bucky. Rotate the patient 20° to the right and centre on the right mid-clavicular line at the level of the lower costal margin.

Collimation for either projection will vary according to the patient's size and shape, as will effective travel of the gallbladder from a midpoint of the liver.

Urinary tract

KIDNEY

Renal area anteroposterior projection
As describe in abdomen – images on arrested inspiration and expiration may be taken to establish the presence of calculi in the renal parenchyma.

Posterior oblique projection
From a supine start rotate the patient 45° towards the side of interest and support with pads. Centre a vertical IR to a point on the rotated midline that lies midway between the xiphisternum and the lower costal margin. Collimate to include the kidney area.

URINARY BLADDER

Axial bladder view
Using a bucky-centred IR angled 20° ↓, centre to a point 7.5 cm superior to the symphysis pubis and collimate to include the whole bladder.

Anterior oblique view
This projection is designed to demonstrate the vesicoureteric junction that is a prime spot for lodging of calculi to cause urinary colic and obstruction.

From a supine position lift the side of interest from the table so the MSP forms an angle of 45° to the image receptor. Centre a vertical IR to a point 5 cm posterior to the rotated midline and 5 cm superior to the symphysis pubis. Collimate to include the whole of the bladder.

SKULL AND CRANIOFACIAL SKELETON EXAMINATIONS

Although of limited use today, some basic skull and facial radiographs have a triage, planning and screening (MRI and orbital metallic foreign body) role to play. Some definitions are helpful to keep in mind:

RBL   radiographic base line = orbitomeatal line (the line joining the outer canthus of the eye to the EAM)

MSP   median sagittal plane = the plane that divides the skull symmetrically in half

ABL   anthropological base line = the line from the infraorbital point to the EAM (also known as Reid's base line)

IOL   interorbital line or IPL (interpupillary line) = a line joining the centre of the two orbits and perpendicular to the MSP

EAM external auditory meatus

Skull

A standard request for skull images would include a 20° OF, a 35° FO (Townes) and either lateral according to side of interest.

OCCIPITOFRONTAL 20° PROJECTION

The patient's head is positioned in true PA with the MSP and RBL perpendicular to the image receptor. Centre in the midline at the glabella with the IR angled 20° ↓ so the petrous ridges are projected to the orbital floors.

FRONTO-OCCIPITAL 35° (TOWNES) PROJECTION

The patient is in the true AP position with RBL and MSP perpendicular to the image receptor. Centre the IR, angled 35° ↓ to a point 5 cm above the nasion. To accommodate the image the receptor may need positioning at shoulder level; conversely, the shoulders may have to be depressed to prevent superimposition and loss of definition of the occipital region.

LATERAL PROJECTION

With the MSP parallel and IPL perpendicular to the image receptor, the patient will be truly lateral. In the seated patient consider shoulder rotation for larger patients to enable the individual to get closer to the receptor without introducing IPL tilting. The image should be obtained so that fluid or air may be detected in the cranial vault so a horizontal IR is required, centred to a point 2.5 cm above the EAM and collimated to the skull and upper cervical spine (C1/2).

FRONTO-OCCIPITAL 10° PROJECTION

This projection can be used in trauma situations to replace the OF 20°. With the patient in a true AP position, MSP and RBL perpendicular to the image receptor, centre the IR angled 10° ↓ to the nasion and collimate to include the whole of the skull.

Facial bones

OCCIPITOMENTAL PROJECTION

In a PA position, rest the patient's nose and chin on the image receptor with the MSP perpendicular and the RBL forming a 45° angle. Centre the IR in the midline at the lower border of the orbits and collimate to include middle and upper one-third of the face. In trauma situations this can be performed by using a vertical IR directed towards a receptor and raising the patient's chin so the RBL is 45° past the vertical relative to the examination table.

30° OCCIPITOMENTAL PROJECTION (OM30)

Use the same positioning as the OM, and centre to the lower orbital margin with a 30° ↓ angulation to the feet. This projection is designed to show the orbital floor but may be used to reveal the zygoma. Similarly a Townes projection collimated to the zygoma with a reduced exposure can produce good results.

LATERAL PROJECTION

Place the head in a true lateral position (MSP parallel and IPL perpendicular to the image receptor) and centre a perpendicular IR 2.5 cm below the outer canthus of the eye. Collimate to include the facial area.

Orbits

OCCIPITOFRONTAL 25° PROJECTION

As for the skull. Ensure the orbital region has no superimposition of the petrous ridges. If for foreign body detection, eye movements may be performed to establish if the FB is present and whether it is anterior or posterior. This is achieved by taking repeat views with the patient looking up then down during exposure +/− looking to one side or the other. A fracture of the orbital floor may be revealed by the 'teardrop' of rectus muscle fat herniating through the bone and allowing air from the maxilla to rise behind and above the globe of the orbit to create the 'black eyebrow sign'.

30° OCCIPITOMENTAL PROJECTION (OM30)

Use the same positioning as the OM centre to the lower orbital margin with a 30° ↓ angulation to the feet. This projection is designed to show the orbital floor for fractures.

LATERAL PROJECTION

As for the facial bones but centre on the outer canthus and collimate to include around the eye only.

Paranasal sinuses

OCCIPITOFRONTAL 20° PROJECTION

The patient's head is positioned in true PA with the MSP and RBL perpendicular to the image receptor. Centre in the midline at the glabella with the IR angled 20° ↓ so the petrous ridges are projected to the orbital floors. Shows the frontal and ethmoidal sinuses.

OCCIPITOMENTAL PROJECTION

In a PA position, rest the patient's nose and chin on the image receptor with the MSP perpendicular and the RBL forming a 45° angle. Centre the IR in the midline at the lower border of the orbits and collimate to include middle and upper thirds of the face. Shows the maxillary sinuses. If fluid is suspected as being present, repeat the image but tilt the head so the IOL is angled 20–25° so that the fluid level will change position.

The OM can also be repeated with an open mouth to project the sphenoid sinus clearly onto the image receptor.

LATERAL PROJECTION

Place the patient's head in a true lateral position (MSP parallel and IPL perpendicular to the image receptor) and centre a perpendicular IR 2.5 cm below the outer canthus of the eye. Collimate to include the facial area so frontal, maxillary and sphenoid sinuses are visualised.

OBLIQUE PROJECTION

Rarely used as CT will better evaluate the posterior ethmoid sinuses. Place the head so that nose, cheek and forehead will rest on the image receptor with MSP 40° and the RBL 30° to the perpendicular. Centre through the orbit in contact with the receptor; reverse the position for the other side.

Mastoid air cells

Rarely imaged today as CT and MRI have taken over.

FRONTO-OCCIPITAL 35° (TOWNES) PROJECTION

The patient is in the true AP position with RBL and MSP perpendicular to the image receptor. Centre the IR in the midline, angled 35° ↓ to pass through the mastoid processes.

LATERAL OBLIQUE PROJECTION

With the patient's head in true lateral position, fold the pinna of the ear forward and use the head to hold it in place against the image receptor. Centre 1.25 cm behind the EAM and take images of both sides for comparison.

Temporomandibular joints

LATERAL OBLIQUE PROJECTION

With the patient's head in true lateral position (MSP parallel and IOL perpendicular to image receptor) centre 5 cm above the EAM away from the film with the IR angled 25° ↓. Take images with the mouth open and closed (back teeth clenched together) to show joint movement relationships.

FRONTO-OCCIPITAL 35° (TOWNES) PROJECTION

The patient is in the true AP position with RBL and MSP perpendicular to the image receptor. Centre the IR in the midline through the EAMs, angled 35° ↓ to the TMJs.

Mandible

POSTEROANTERIOR PROJECTION

The patient is prone or erect in the PA skull position with mouth slightly open and IR perpendicular to the image receptor. Centre 6 cm below the RBL and collimate to include the heads of mandible and symphysis menti.

LATERAL PROJECTION

The patient's head is in the true lateral position and IR perpendicular to the image receptor. Centre midway between the EAM and symphysis menti. Collimate to include the whole mandible and soft tissues.

OBLIQUE PROJECTION

Position the patient's head truly lateral and place the side of interest against the receptor. Angle the IR 25° ↑ relative to the mandible and centre 5 cm below the angle of the jaw, collimating to include the whole mandible. Alternatively, with an IR perpendicular to the film, tilt the head so the MSP is at 25° to the receptor. Centre 5 cm below the angle of the mandible.

Chapter 4

Named Radiography Projections

Definitions

METHOD

A radiographic position or procedure named after the person who developed it.

PROJECTION

The direction or path of the X-ray beam as it passes through the patient.

VIEW

The finished radiograph or image of the relevant anatomy.

INDEX

ABDOMEN

Butterfly – rectosigmoid
Hamptons – rectosigmoid

ANKLE

Mortise – AP with 15–20° medial rotation

CHEST

Flying angel view – thoracic inlet
Lindbölm – AP lordotic
Williams method – costovertebral and costotransverse joints

Index of Medical Imaging, First Edition. Jonathan McConnell.
© 2011 Blackwell Publishing Ltd. Published 2011 by Blackwell Publishing Ltd.

ELBOW

Berquist – capitellum – radial head fracture
Capitellum projection
Coyle trauma methods – radial head, coronoid process of ulna
Jones – flexion elbow
Laquerriere and Pierquin method – supero-inferior ulnar groove
Pierquin method – supero-inferior ulnar groove
Tomas and Proubasta – radial head
Tuberosity view – elbow
Veihwëger method – ulnar groove projection

FOOT

Anthonson – subtalar joints
Broden I and II – subtalar joints
Causton method – sesamoids
Coalition – calcaneotalar coalition
Feist-Mankin subtalar joints (see also Isherwood method)
Grashey – prone, oblique
Harris – subtalar, coalition
Harris and Beam – calcaneum
Harris-Beath method – middle subtalar joint
Holly – AP sesamoids
Isherwood method – subtalar joints
Kandel – clubfoot
Kite – clubfoot
Lewis – PA sesamoids
Lilienfeld – calcaneum
Lunge position – weight-bearing lateral foot
Prayer position – lateral calcanei
Schuss – weight-bearing lateral foot
Simmons – talipes equinovarus (clubfoot)
Talar neck view – oblique foot

HAND AND WRIST

Ball catcher – AP oblique hand
Betts – first carpometacarpal joint
Brewerton – metacarpal heads
Bridgeman – scaphoid
Burman – first carpometacarpal joint

Carpal boss – carpometacarpal joint
Carpal bridge – tangential carpus
Carpal canal projection
Daffner, Emmerling and Buterbaugh – scaphoid and capitate
Gaynor-Hart – carpal tunnel
Lentino – carpal bridge
Lewis – AP thumb
Long and Rafert – AP thumb
Norgaard method – AP oblique
Rafert-Long – scaphoid
Robert – AP thumb
Stecher – scaphoid
Templeton and Zim – carpal tunnel
Ziter method – scaphoid

KNEE

Ahlback – AP weight-bearing
Beclére – intercondylar
Brattstrom – skyline/tangential patella
Camp Coventry – intercondylar, prone
Ficat – skyline seated, tangential patella tracking views
Frik – intercondylar
Holmblad – intercondylar
Hughston – prone tangential patella
Jaroschy-Hughston – tangential patella for subluxation
Kuchendorf – PA oblique patella
Laurin's – tangential patella
Merchant – tangential patella
Rosenberg – PA weight-bearing, flexed patella
Settegast – tangential patella
Skyline – tangential patella
Sunrise – tangential patella

MAMMOGRAPHY

Eklund technique

PELVIS AND HIP

Charnley
Cleaves – axial, frog leg
Clements Nakayama – lateral hip

Colonna – acetabulum
Danelius-Miller – horizontal beam hip
Danelius-Miller modification or Lorenz method – see above
Dunlap, Swanson and Penner method – acetabula in profile
False profile view = Lequesne method – erect hip
Ferguson – sacro-iliac joints
Flamingo – erect symphysis pubis
Friedman – oblique hip
Frog-leg – lateral hip
Hickey – mediolateral hip
Inlet and outlet views – pelvic trauma
Johnson – axiolateral hip
Judet – acetabulum
Kisch method – oblique hip
Lauenstein – frog lateral
Lauenstein and Hickey method – mediolateral hip
Leonard-George method – supine with curved cassette
Lequesne – erect hip
Letournel – iliac wing
Lilienfeld – acetabulum and symphysis pubis
Lowenstein method – frog leg lateral hips
Modified Cleave's – bilateral frog leg
Pennal's method (Tile's method) – inlet and outlet pelvic trauma
Penner – acetabulum (= Swanson, Dunlap)
Risser – iliac epiphysis
Sanderson – mediolateral oblique hip
Schneider – femoral head
Staunig – pubic and ischial bones
Stork – like flamingo – symphysis pubis
Sven-Johannson – horizontal beam lateral hip
Swanson – acetabulum (= Dunlap, Penner)
Taylor – pubic and ischial bones
Teufel – acetabulum and femoral head margin
Tile's method – inlet and outlet views pelvic trauma
Urist's method – acetabular rim (see Lequesne method)

SHOULDER, CLAVICLE AND ACROMIOCLAVICULAR JOINT

Adams – prone
Alexander – acromioclavicular joint
Alexander stress method – acromioclavicular joint

Bigliani's classification – outlet view; see Neer
Blackett-Healy – prone tangential
Didiée view – prone
Fisk – bicipital groove
Garth – trauma dislocation
Grashy – true AP
Hermodsson's – internal rotation and tangential
Hill-Sachs defect – impaction fracture of humeral head
Johner – supine tangential
Laquerriere and Pierquin – supine scapula
Lawrence – proximal humerus, transthoracic
Miller – query dislocation
Neer – outlet
Oppenheim – cephaloscapular projection
Outlet view – for humeral impingement
Pearson – acromioclavicular joint
Quesada – clavicle prone
Stryker – posterior humeral head
Supraspinatus outlet view – acromion
Tarrant – clavicle
Wallace-Hellier – AP
West Point view – glenoid rim – prone
Y view – axial shoulder or lateral scapula
Zanca's view – acromioclavicular joint

SKULL, SINUSES AND FACIAL BONES

Albers-Schonberg – temporomandibular joint
Bertel – orbital floors
Blondeau – occiptomental facial bones
Caldwell – occiptofrontal
Grashey – see Townes
Hääs – petrous temporal
Henkeltopf – zygomatic arches
Hirtz – submento vertex
Jug handle view – submento vertex zygomatic arches
Macqueen-Dell – mandibular condyle
May view – zygomatic arch
Modified Townes – condyloid process of mandible
Pirie – occiptomental sinus view, mouth open
Reverse Caldwell – AP

Reverse Townes – PA Townes skull
Reverse Waters –AP facial bones
Titterington – occiptomental 30° view
Townes – AP axial skull
Townes (modified) – condylar process of mandible
Waters – sinuses occiptomental projection, reverse Waters
Zanelli method – temporomandibular joints, open and closed

SPINE

Duncan-Hoew – flexion, extension lumbar spine
Ferguson method – scoliosis
Ferguson's view – sacro-iliac joints
Fuch – odontoid
Grandy – lateral cervical spine
Judd – odontoid
Kasabach – odontoid
Kovacs – lumbar spine
Monda – cervicothoracic junction
Otonello method – moving jaw, AP cervical spine
Pawlow method – C7/T1
Pillar views – cervical spine
Risser – iliac crests
Twining – C7/T1
Swimmer's projection

STERNOCLAVICULAR JOINTS

Heinig – horizontal beam lateral
Hobb – PA
Kurzbauer – lateral
Serendipity – query dislocation

NAMED PROJECTIONS

ADAMS' SHOULDER METHOD

Patient is supine with the humerus horizontal to the top of the table. Arm adducted to the side of the patient, the humerus is internally rotated 70–100°, with forearm alongside the hip. IR 15° ↓ to the humeral head with 18 × 24 cm image receptor placed beneath the shoulder.

AHLBACK METHOD

Weight-bearing AP view of the knee in full extension. Centre a horizontal IR midway between the knees on a single image receptor. Discussed as Leach, Gregg and Siber in *REF: Frank et al. 2007a p. 308*

ALBERS-SCHÖNBERG

Demonstrates the TMJs. True lateral head with IR 20° ↑ to TMJ closest to film. Use 18 × 24 cm image receptor.

ALEXANDER METHOD (ACROMIOCLAVICULAR JOINT)

Routine axial oblique view of the acromioclavicular joint. Projects ACJ superiorly compared with standard AP projection. AP or PA. IR 15° ↑ to coracoid process on 18 × 24 cm receptor – process as detail. *REF: Frank et al. 2007a pp. 204–205*

ALEXANDER STRESS METHOD

PA axial oblique projection of the acromioclavicular joint. Shows PA axial oblique image of ACJ relative to other bones of shoulder.

Position as for lateral scapula (RAO or LAO). Patient is then asked to thrust the affected shoulder forward, reaching the hand across to opposite axilla. IR 15° ↓ through ACJ. *REF: Frank et al. 2007a pp. 206–207*

ANTHONSON'S METHOD

Subtalar joint projection. Foot in the lateral position. Dorsiflex the foot. IR 25° to the ankle and 30° around the vertical axis of the X-ray tube column to the toes. Centre immediately below the medial malleolus. *REF: Ballinger & Frank 1999a p. 268*

BALL CATCHER'S VIEW

See NORGAARD METHOD.

BECLÉRE METHOD

View of the intercondylar fossa in profile.

Patient is supine. Knee flexed so that the long axis of the femur forms an angle of 120° to the long axis of the tibia. Image receptor under knee. IR at right angles to the long axis of the tibia 1.5 cm below apex of patella. Similar to Friks method. *REF: Frank et al. 2007a p. 316; Bontrager & Lampignano 2010 pp. 251–253*

BERTEL

Demonstrates the orbital floors and the infraorbital fissure.

Head in the PA position with radiographic baseline at right angles to the film. Centre IR to the nasion with the tube angled 20°↑. *REF: Goldman & Cope 1993; Ballinger & Frank 1999a p. 298*

BETT'S PROJECTION

Also known as Clements Nakayama projection of thumb.

PA axial oblique to demonstrate the thumb, carpometacarpal, trapezium-second metacarpal, trapezium-trapezoid and scapho-trapezial joints.

The patient sits parallel with the long axis of the table, forearm resting on the image receptor. From a lateral wrist position rotate hand anteriorly onto a 45° pad. Use ulnar deviation to achieve a position whereby the first metacarpal is parallel with the image receptor. Angle the IR 45° along the long axis of the metacarpal and collimate to include the area suggested above. *REF: Frank et al. 2007a p. 136*

BIGLIANI'S CLASSIFICATION SYSTEM

Radiological assessment of acromial morphology using supraspinatus outlet radiographs (Y projection); see NEER METHOD.

BLACKETT-HEALY METHOD

A tangential projection of the insertion of the teres minor or subscapularis tendons.

Teres minor: Patient is prone. Place image receptor under the shoulder. Abduct the arm, flex the elbow, and internally rotate the arm so the back of the hand rests on the lumbosacral region of the back. Centre to the humeral head, IR at 90° to receptor. *REF: Ballinger & Frank 1999a p. 188*

Subscapularis: Patient is supine. Abduct the arm, flex the elbow, and pronate the hand. Centre to the shoulder joint, IR at 90° to receptor. *REF: Ballinger & Frank 1999a p. 189*

BLONDEAU

Routine OM facial bones (Waters projection) with radiographic baseline overtilted by 5°. *REF: Frank et al. 2007a p. 354; Bontrager & Lampignano 2010 p. 422 (modified Waters)*

BRATTSTRÖM METHOD

Skyline projections of patellae to demonstrate intercondylar sulcus angle in patients with recurrent dislocations. Both knees for comparison.

1 Merchant method – to evaluate subluxation. Relaxation of the quadriceps femoris muscles is critical.
2 Laurin's method – with 20° flexion at the knee to measure lateral patellofemoral angle.
3 Stress axilla view – made with knee flexed off end of table and constant lateral pressure to patella in an attempt to displace patella laterally. Comparison made with asymptomatic knees.
4 Sunrise projection – tangential view of patella. Patient is prone, knee flexed to 115°. IR 15° towards the apex of patella along axis of tibia and fibula.

REF: http://www.wheelessonline.com/ortho/axilla_view_of_the_patella

BREWERTON'S METHOD

Demonstrates erosions of the metacarpal heads and the bases of the phalanges.

Hand in the AP position, i.e. palm up. The metacarpophalangeal joints are flexed to 45° with the phalanges in contact with the film. Tube angled 20° → (IR from ulnar side) to the head of the third metacarpal. *REF: Dye 2009*

BRIDGEMAN VIEW

See also STECHER METHOD 1.
To elongate the scaphoid to reveal subtle fractures.

PA wrist position with the image receptor inclined by 20° so that the hand is higher than the wrist. Centre to the scaphoid. *REF: Frank et al. 2007a pp. 132–133; Bontrager & Lampignano 2010 p. 156*

BRODEN I (MEDIAL ROTATION)

Subtalar joint view demonstrating posterior articulation.

Foot positioned as for AP ankle, then rotate the foot 45° medially. Angle the tube ↑ so IR is 10, 20, 30 and 40° to the subtalar joint. Similar to ISHERWOOD METHOD but with more angulation positions. *REF: Frank et al. 2007a p. 283*

BRODEN II (LATERAL ROTATION)

Subtalar joint view.

Foot positioned as for AP ankle, then rotate the foot 45° externally (lateral rotation). Angle the tube ↑ so IR is 15° to the subtalar joint. *REF: Frank et al. 2007a p. 284*

BURMAN

To demonstrate the first carpometacarpal joint.

Seat patient at the end of the table and extend the forearm to lie parallel with the long axis of the image receptor. Hyperextend the hand (a bandage around the fingers may be used to maintain the position) and rotate internally so the lateral border (radial side) of the thumb is flat on the image receptor. IR 45° along the CMC joint towards the elbow. *REF: Frank et al. 2007a pp. 112–113*

BUTTERFLY VIEWS

Elongated views of the rectosigmoid segments of large intestine.

AP butterfly: Centre 5 cm inferior to the anterior-superior iliac spine (ASIS) and angle the vertical IR 40° ↑.

LPO butterfly: Centre 5 cm inferiorly to and 5 cm medially to the right ASIS. Angle the vertical central ray 40° ↑.

PA butterfly: Centre to the ASIS and angle the vertical central ray 40° ↓.

RAO butterfly: Centre to the level of the ASIS and 5 cm to the left of the lumbar spinous processes. Angle the vertical central ray 40° ↓.

REF: Ballinger & Frank 1999b pp. 138–147; Bontrager & Lampignano 2010 pp. 523–524

CALDWELL METHOD

PA axial projection of the skull.
IR 15°↓ to radiographic base line (RBL) centred to exit at nasion. *REF: Frank et al. 2007b pp. 358–359; Bontrager & Lampignano 2010 p. 394 (cranium), p. 421 (sinuses)*

REVERSE CALDWELL

AP projection of the skull.
Angle IR 15°↑ to RBL. Useful for trauma patients. *REF: Bontrager & Lampignano 2010 pp. 620–621*

CAMP COVENTRY METHOD

View of the intercondylar notch.
Patient is prone. The tibia is elevated to form an angle of 40–50° relative to the examination table. The IR is directed ↓ to the knee joint so that it makes a right angle with the long axis of the tibia. *REF: Frank et al. 2007a pp. 314–315; Bontrager & Lampignano 2010 pp. 249–250*

CAPITELLUM PROJECTION (BERQUIST METHOD)

View to demonstrate fractures of the radial head.
Patient positioned as for lateral elbow. The IR is angled 45° to the forearm parallel with the humeral axis. Centre to the radial head. *REF: Ballinger & Frank 1999a p. 141*

CARPAL BOSS

Demonstrates bony protuberance on the dorsum of the wrist (os styloideum) at the level of the second and third carpometacarpal joints.
From a lateral wrist starting point, supinate the wrist 30° and slightly ulnar deviate. This places the dorsal prominence at the dorsoradial aspect of the second to third carpometacarpal joints at a tangent to the vertical IR. Centre IR to pass through the dorsal prominence. *REF: Conway et al. 1985*

Named Radiography Projections

CARPAL BRIDGE VIEW

A tangential projection of the carpus to particularly demonstrate fractures of the scaphoid, lunate dislocations, and foreign bodies in the dorsum of the wrist.

The patient stands with their back towards the examination table. The palm of the hand rests on the image receptor with the forearm at right angles to the hand. Direct the central ray 4 cm proximal to the wrist joint with a 45° angle ↓ towards the fingers. Demonstrated as a modified version in *REF: Frank et al. 2007a p. 137 fig. 4:97*

CARPAL CANAL PROJECTION

A projection to demonstrate the carpal canal made up of the palmar aspect of the trapezium, scaphoid tuberosity, trapezoid and capitate, the hamulus process of the hamate, the triquetrum and the pisiform. Also termed GAYNOR-HART METHOD.

Inferosuperior carpal tunnel projection. Position patient at end of table with forearm (PA) parallel with long axis of table. Hyperextend wrist, holding fingers back. Centre 5 cm distal to the base of the third metacarpal, angle IR 25–30° from the vertical to meet the long axis of the hand and travel along the carpal tunnel. *REF: Frank et al. 2007a pp. 138–139; Bontrager & Lampignano 2010 p. 158*

CAUSTON METHOD

Oblique foot projection to demonstrate the sesamoids.

Foot is lateral with the medial side against the image receptor. Angle the IR 40° towards the ankle and centre to the first metatarsophalangeal sesamoids. *REF: Frank et al. 2007a p. 254*

CHARNLEY'S METHOD

AP pelvis. IR centred on symphysis pubis with field collimated to include all of a hip prosthesis.

CLEAVES METHOD (HIP)

Axial projection of the femoral heads, necks and trochanteric areas projected onto one film.

Position as a frog-leg lateral and centre to the symphysis pubis with the IR angled to be parallel with the long axes of the femoral shafts. Approx 40°↑. *REF: Frank et al. 2007a p. 352*

MODIFIED CLEAVES METHOD: as above without IR angulation – may also be employed for a single hip projection. *REF: Frank et al. 2007a p. 350*

CLEMENTS NAKAYAMA METHOD

Modified axiolateral view of the acetabulum and femoral head.

This method can be used where the opposite hip cannot be raised for a horizontal beam lateral hip. Patient is supine, with the affected side near the table edge, position the film vertically and parallel to the neck of femur. IR directed across opposite thigh with 15°↓ angle from horizontal but perpendicular to femoral neck and image receptor. *REF: Frank et al. 2007a p. 360*

COALITION PROJECTION

Demonstrates a calcaneotalar coalition.

Patient stands with the image receptor under the long axis of the calcaneum. Angle the IR 45° from vertical to direct it through the posterior surface of the flexed ankle to the level of the base of the fifth metatarsal. *REF: Frank et al. 2007a p. 279*

COLONNA METHOD

A projection that demonstrates the slope of the acetabular roof and the depth of the socket.

Patient lies on unaffected side. Unaffected leg extended in true lateral position. Flex knee of affected side and support. Rotate patient's pelvis 15–17°, enough to separate the projection of the hip joints. IR is perpendicular to image receptor through affected hip. *REF: Ballinger & Frank 1999a p. 356*

COYLE TRAUMA METHODS

Projections of the radial head and/or the coronoid process of the ulna.

Radial head view: Elbow flexed 90° and hand pronated. Angle the IR 45° → the elbow towards the shoulder. Centre to the radial head. Reverse direction to CAPITELLUM PROJECTION (wrist lateral).

Coronoid process view: Elbow flexed 80° from extended position with the hand pronated. Angle the IR 45° → away from the shoulder (along axis of humerus) and directed to the elbow joint. *REF: Coyle 1980; Frank et al. 2007a pp. 154–156; Bontrager & Lampignano 2010 pp. 168–169*

DAFFNER, EMMERLING AND BUTERBAUGH METHOD

Projections to elongate scaphoid and capitate.

Position as for PA wrist with IR 30° from vertical towards the carpal bones. Angle toward elbow to elongate both scaphoid and capitate and toward metacarpals to elongate capitate only. *REF: Frank et al. 2007a p. 133 (variation on Stecher's view of scaphoid and capitate)*

DANELIUS-MILLER METHOD

Routine horizontal beam axiolateral (inferosuperior) projection of the hip.

Place an image receptor with grid at 45° to the lateral border of the pelvis on the affected side. Flex the knee and hip to elevate the unaffected leg and support. Direct a horizontal IR beneath the elevated limb so it is perpendicular to the image receptor. Collimate accordingly. *REF: Frank et al. 2007a pp. 358–359; Bontrager 1997 p. 239*

DANELIUS-MILLER MODIFICATION OR LORENZ METHOD

Similar to DANELIUS-MILLER METHOD but used where the patient is unable to fully flex the hip or knee of the unaffected side.

Elevate the unaffected leg as far as possible so it will be outside the radiation field and support. Establish the centring point in the femoral neck using the bisector of the line between ASIS and symphysis pubis extended 2.5 cm inferiorly. Centre the IR to the image receptor placed alongside the femoral neck as described for the DANELIUS-MILLER METHOD. *REF: Skripkus & Gentili 2006 p. 13*

DIDIÉE METHOD

Shoulder projection for humeral head defects.

Patient is prone with cassette under the shoulder. Humerus parallel to the table top with a 7.5 cm pad under the elbow.

Forearm behind trunk of body with dorsum of hand on the iliac crest, thumb directed upward. IR angled 45°↓ centred on the glenohumeral joint. A modified projection is achieved with the same position of patient and IR but further angulation of the IR 45° lateromedially towards the head of the humerus. *REF: Long & Rafert 1995 pp. 174–175*

DUNCAN-HOEW METHOD

Flexion and extension views of the lumbar spine.

Patient is laid on the table in right or left lateral decubitus position and asked to hyperflex and hyperextend. A vertical IR centred to the bucky is used with collimation to cover the area taken by the patient. May also be performed erect when examining for weight-bearing effects. *REF: Frank et al. 2007a pp. 456–457 (but not named)*

DUNLAP, SWANSON AND PENNER METHOD

Projection to show the acetabulae in profile.

The patient is sat upright on the bucky table with their legs over the side. The vertical central ray is directed 30° towards the lateral aspect of the pelvis towards the acetabulum. *REF: Ballinger & Frank 1999a p. 3*

EKLUND TECHNIQUE

Mammography technique for patients with implants. These extra views of the breast with the implant 'pinched' back demonstrate the anterior breast tissue, in the CC and MLO positions. *REF: Bontrager & Lampignano 2010 p. 579*

FALSE PROFILE VIEW

Gives a view of the acetabulum in profile. Alternative view with patient supine is URIST'S METHOD.

See the LEQUESNE METHOD for positioning.

FEIST-MANKIN METHOD

To show subtalar joints. See the ISHERWOOD METHOD.

FERGUSON METHOD (FOR SCOLIOSIS)

Demonstrates the thoracic and lumbar spine in the AP projection and identifies the deforming (primary) curve from the compensatory curve. Two films are taken, one standing erect AP and one with the foot or hip on the convex side of the curve elevated. *REF: Frank et al. 2007a pp. 452–453; Bontrager & Lampignano 2010 p. 340*

FERGUSON'S VIEW (FOR SACRO-ILIAC JOINTS)

View of the sacro-iliac joints and lumbosacral junction. With this projection, the symphysis pubis overlaps the sacrum but helps in evaluating injury to the sacral bones, the pubis and the ischial rami.

The patient is in the same position as for the AP pelvis. The tube in angled between 30° ↑ (♂) and 35° ↑ (♀) and is centred to the mid-portion of the pelvis. It shows the SI joints more clearly. *REF: Frank et al. 2007a pp. 436–438*

FICAT METHOD

Axial patella projection to demonstrate patella dislocations/ subluxations during tracking.

Patient on table with knee flexed 25–30° with and without external rotation of tibia. Centre IR tangential to patella with incident receptor supported on the femur so the superior aspect of patella is closest. Repeated with knee also flexed at 60 and 90°. X-ray tube points from feet towards chest of patient. Similar to HUGHSTON that has been inverted. *REF: Frank et al. 2007a pp. 324–325; Bontrager & Lampignano 2010 pp. 255–256; emedicine.com/ sports/topic95htm*

FISK METHOD

A projection of the bicipital groove.

The patient is erect. Flex the elbow and lean patient across the table with the 24 × 30 image receptor resting on the forearm and in the crook of the elbow while the hand is supinated. Centre IR to the bicipital groove and suspend respiration for exposure. *REF: Frank et al. 2007a pp. 200–201; Fisk 1965*

FLAMINGO METHOD

Stress views of the symphysis pubis to evaluate residual subluxation following previous injury.

Two views. Patient stands on each leg in turn. Centre to the symphysis pubis. *REF: Anderson et al. 1998 p.148*

FLYING ANGEL

Routine lateral thoracic inlet projection. *REF: Ballinger & Frank 1999a p. 521 (not named); Ballinger & Frank 1999b p. 30 (soft palate, pharynx and larynx); Bontrager & Lampignano 2010 p. 99*

FRIEDMAN METHOD

Axiolateral projection of femoral head, neck and upper femur.

Roll the patient towards the affected side. Position leg in lateral position. IR 35° ↑ to midfemoral neck. Kisch recommends the central ray be angled 20° ↑. *REF: Ballinger & Frank 1999a p. 352*

FRIK'S METHOD

AP projection of intercondylar notch. See BECLÉRE METHOD.

FROG-LEG POSITION (MODIFIED CLEAVES, LAUENSTEIN AND HICKEY METHODS)

AP oblique projection of both hips, particularly to evaluate comparatively for slipped upper femoral epiphysis.

Patient is supine with the knees flexed and legs abducted so the soles of the feet are in contact. Ensure the femora are matched in their positions relative to the top of the examination table. Centre the IR perpendicular to image receptor at a point 2.5 cm superior to symphysis pubis. *REF: Frank et al. 2007a p. 350; Bontrager & Lampignano 2010 p. 270*

FUCH'S METHOD

AP projection for dens (C2 peg) within foramen magnum.

The patient is supine on the examination table. Extend the chin until symphysis menti and mastoids tips (mentomeatal line;

MML) is perpendicular to table top. The IR should be parallel to MML at tip of chin midway between mastoid tips. *REF: Frank et al. 2007a p. 392; Bontrager & Lampignano 2010 p. 313*

GARTH METHOD

May also be termed MILLER'S METHOD.

Apical axial oblique view of the shoulder, useful for trauma dislocation cases.

Centre to the head of the humerus. Patient is erect or supine rotated 45° to the affected side, central ray angled 45° ↓. If the head of the humerus is projected below the glenoid then the dislocation is anterior. If the head of the humerus is projected above the glenoid then the dislocation is posterior. *REF: Bontrager & Lampignano 2010 pp. 198–199*

GAYNOR-HART METHOD

Inferosuperior carpal tunnel projection.

Position patient at end of table with forearm (PA) parallel with long axis of table. Hyperextend wrist, holding fingers back with bandage or other hand. Centre IR 5 cm distal to the base of the third metacarpal (palmar aspect), angle 25–30° from the vertical to the long axis of the hand. *REF: Frank et al. 2007a pp. 138–139; Bontrager & Lampignano 2010 p. 158*

See also TEMPLETON AND ZIM METHOD.

GRANDY METHOD

Routine lateral cervical spine with deliberate rolling forwards or back of the shoulders, depending on the natural position of the patient, to reveal whole of cervical spine. Use a horizontal IR centred on C4, chin slightly elevated and coronal plane of the head and neck perpendicular to image receptor. Collimate to include all cervical spine to T1. *REF: Frank et al. 2007a pp. 400–401*

GRASHEY METHOD (SHOULDER)

Routine view of the shoulder to demonstrate the glenohumeral joint space.

Rotate patient 35–45° until scapula is parallel to film. Slightly abduct arm. Neutral rotation of humerus. Centre IR to scapulo-humeral joint. *REF: Frank et al. 2007a pp. 192–193; Bontrager & Lampignano 2010 p. 190*

GRASHEY METHOD (SKULL)

Patient positioned as for AP skull with the OM baseline perpendicular to film. IR 30° ↓ and centre between the upper borders of the EAMs.

See TOWNES PROJECTION.

GRASHEY METHODS (FOOT)

Oblique plantodorsal projections of the foot.
Patient is prone, dorsal surface of foot in contact with receptor. Centre vertical IR to the base of the third metatarsal.

1 To demonstrate the space between the first and second metatarsals, rotate the heel medially 30°.
2 To demonstrate the spaces between the second and third, the third and fourth, and the fourth and fifth metatarsals, adjust the foot so that the heel is rotated laterally 20°.

REF: Ballinger & Frank 1999a p. 248

HÄÄS METHOD (REVERSE TOWNES)

Patient PA without rotation. OML perpendicular to film. IR 25° ↑ 3.5 cm below inion passing through at level of EAMs. *REF: Frank et al. 2007a p. 322; Bontrager & Lampignano 2010 p. 397*

HAMPTONS PROJECTION

Demonstrates sigmoid colon during barium enema examinations.
Patient is prone with ASIS equidistant from table top. Angle IR 30–35° ↓ and centre to the first sacral segment. See also BUTTERFLY VIEWS for further variations of this region. *REF: Carver & Carver 2006 p. 419*

HARRIS METHOD

Axial projection of the heel. Useful for demonstrating talocalcaneal bars.

Patient stands with both feet on the film. The patient leans forward slightly. The tube is positioned behind the patient and the central ray is angled 45° towards the heels and is centred between the medial malleoli. Described using 40° angulation but not named; similar to LILIENFELD METHOD. *REF: Frank et al. 2007a p. 279*

HARRIS AND BEAM (SKI JUMP)

Three axial projections of the calcaneum (both sides).

Patient standing, tube positioned behind the patient, central ray centred between the feet and then angled 35, 40 and 45° towards the calcaneum as in HARRIS METHOD and HARRIS-BEATH METHOD.

HARRIS-BEATH METHOD

Axial view of calcaneum but taken with the patient prone; foot dorsiflexed and slightly internally rotated. To demonstrate primarily middle facet of the subtalar joint, but also the posterior facet and is particularly useful in the diagnosis of talocalcaneal coalition or fracture of the sustentaculum tali. *REF: Anderson et al. 1998 pp. 298–299*

A similar projection without the emphasis on internal rotation is described in *REF: Ballinger & Frank 1999a p. 264*

HEINIG METHOD

Horizontal beam projection of sternoclavicular joints.

Patient is supine with cassette supported beside patient on uninvolved side. CR tangential to the joint and parallel to opposite clavicle at sternoclavicular junction. *REF: Bucholz et al. 2010 p. 1247*

HENKELTOPF METHOD

Routine inferosuperior view of the zygomatic arches (jug handles). Submentovertex projection. No head rotation. IOML

parallel to film. IR midway between zygomatic arches, perpendicular to film. *DO NOT* use immediately following trauma –
suggest use of a TOWNES PROJECTION to prevent hyperextension
neck injury. *REF: Frank et al. 2007a pp. 362–363*

HERMODSSON'S METHOD (INTERNAL ROTATION VIEW)

Shoulder view for subscapular insertion.

Patient is supine with the humerus horizontal to the top of the
table. Arm adducted to the side of the patient, the humerus is
internally rotated 45°, the forearm lies across the anterior trunk.
IR 15° ↓ and centred over the humeral head. *REF: Bucholz et al.
2006 p. 1231*

A similar projection, without angulation, is described in *REF:
Ballinger & Frank 1999a p. 189*

HERMODSSON'S METHOD (TANGENTIAL)

Shoulder projection.

Patient is prone. The elbow is flexed 90° and the dorsum of the
hand is placed behind the trunk, over the upper lumbar spine.
The thumb points upward. The film is placed superior to the
adducted arm. The X-ray tube is placed posterior, lateral and
inferior to the elbow joint, making a 30° angle with the humeral
axis. *REF: Rockwood et al. 1996 p. 1231*

HICKEY METHOD

Mediolateral projection of hip with 20–25° angulation ↑ to project
the femoral neck free of superimposition by the greater trochanter.
Similar to DANELIUS-MILLER METHOD with angulation as
described. *REF: Frank et al. 2007a p. 358*

See LAUENSTEIN METHOD.

HILL-SACHS FRACTURE OR DEFECT VIEW

See LAWRENCE METHOD. This is the Rafert modification of the
inferosuperior axiolateral projection of shoulder performed *as
follow-up* to reveal effects of trauma.

Position as for inferosuperior shoulder with arm in extreme external rotation. The thumb is pointing down and posteriorly so hand is at a 45° oblique angle. Place image receptor so it is parallel with superior surface of shoulder and with a horizontal IR angled 15° medially (aimed at acromioclavicular joint); collimate to include glenohumeral joint. *REF: Frank et al. 2007a pp. 182–183*

HIRTZ METHOD

The routine SMV projection.

Described but named as 'Schuller' in *REF: Frank et al. 2007a pp. 324–325; Bontrager & Lampignano 2010 p. 396*

DO NOT use the SMV method immediately following trauma due to increased hyperextension injury risk to the neck.

HOBB'S METHOD

PA projection of both sternoclavicular joints for query dislocation.

The patient sits at the end of the examination table to lean over the image receptor so the lower thorax is against it. The elbows are rested either side of the receptor on the table to support the patient. The neck is flexed so it is almost parallel with the table top. Centre a vertical IR to the manubrium of sternum and collimate to include both sternoclavicular joints. *REF: Cope 1993; Bucholz et al. 2010 p. 1248*

AP projection: see SERENDIPITY METHOD.

HOLLY METHOD

Views of the sesamoid bones of the first metatarsal.

Patient is supine with heel against cassette. Foot held in dorsiflexion. IR perpendicular and tangential to first metatarsophalangeal joint. *REF: Frank et al. 2007a pp. 252–253*

HÖLMBLAD METHOD

PA intercondylar view of the knee.

Patient on X-ray table kneels 'on all fours' and leans forward 20–30°. The lower leg lies on the table. Centre to the posterior skin crease of the knee. May be done with patient standing or resting a knee on a stool. *REF: Frank et al. 2007a pp. 312–313; Bontrager & Lampignano 2010 pp. 249–251*

HUGHSTON METHOD

Tangential patella projection.

Patient is prone. Knee flexed to 55°. IR 15–20° from long axis of lower leg tangential to patellofemoral joint (PFJ) so IR passes through the PFJ inferosuperiorly. *REF: Frank et al. 2007a p. 321; Bontrager & Lampignano 2010 pp. 255–257*

INLET AND OUTLET VIEWS (PELVIS)

See PENNAL'S METHOD.

ISHERWOOD METHODS (SUBTALAR REGION)

1 Projection to demonstrate the anterior subtalar articulation. Medial border of the foot at a 45° angle to the image receptor. Centre 2.5 cm distal and 2.5 cm anterior to the lateral malleolus.
2 Projection to demonstrate the middle articulation of the subtalar joint and give an 'end-on' view of the sinus tarsi. Foot in the AP ankle position. Rotate the ankle 30° medially. Centre IR to a point 2.5 cm distal and 2.5 cm anterior to the lateral malleolus with a 10° ↑ angulation.
3 Projection to demonstrate the posterior articulation of the subtalar joint in profile. Foot in the AP ankle position. Rotate the ankle 30° laterally. Centre to a point 2.5 cm distal to the medial malleolus with a 10° ↑ angulation.

REF: Frank et al. 2007a pp. 282–284

JAROSCHY METHOD

Patella view. See HUGHSTON METHOD.

JOHNER METHOD

Tangential shoulder view.

Patient is supine with the elbow flexed and the forearm resting on the abdomen. Film placed vertically against the superior

Named Radiography Projections

aspect of the shoulder. Angle the central ray 20° medially and 20° below the horizontal. Centre to the head of the humerus.

JOHNSON METHOD

An axiolateral projection of the femoral head and neck.

Patient in the AP pelvis position. Place the cassette vertically against the lateral aspect of the hip of interest. Tilt the image receptor backward 25°. Direct the horizontal central ray 25° ↓ to match the image receptor angle and rotate the X-ray tube 25° to centre to the femoral neck. *REF: Johnson 1932*

Similar to CLEMENTS NAKAYAMA METHOD but with greater angulation. *REF: Frank et al. 2007a pp. 360–361*

JONES POSITION

View of the elbow in flexion to demonstrate the olecranon process in profile and the distal humerus. May be used where patient refuses to extend the elbow.

Place the humerus on the image receptor and flex the arm. Two projections taken, one with the central ray angled at right angles to the forearm (for olecranon) and another with the central ray angled at right angles to the humerus (for distal humerus). *REF: Bontrager & Lampignano 2010 p. 167 (described but not named); Ballinger & Frank 1999a pp. 138–139*

JUDD METHOD

PA projection of C1–2 (dens) through foramen magnum. Patient PA with MML perpendicular to image receptor. IR parallel to MML through mid-occipital bone, inferoposterior to mastoid tips. *REF: Bontrager 1997 p. 273*

JUDET METHOD

AP oblique projection (RPO and LPO) of the acetabulum.

1 Raise the affected side up by 45° (internal oblique).
2 Raise the unaffected side by 45° (external oblique).

In both cases centre perpendicular IR to the acetabulum of the affected side and adjust exposure in recognition of body part relative to image receptor. *REF: Frank et al. 2007a pp. 364–366; Bontrager 1997 p. 237*

JUG HANDLE PROJECTION

SMV projection of the zygomatic arches.

1 Bilateral. IOML parallel to film. Centre IR perpendicular to receptor midway between zygomatic arches. *REF: Frank et al. 2007b p. 363; Bontrager & Lampignano 2010 p. 396*
2 Unilateral (tangential view). IOML parallel to receptor. Rotate 15° towards side being examined and chin 15° toward side of interest (top of head away from side of interest). Centre IR to zygomatic arch of interest, perpendicular to film and IOML

KANDEL METHOD

Superoplantar projection to demonstrate clubfoot.
  The patient stands on the cassette. The vertical IR is angled 40° and directed to the heel so that it emerges from the midfoot. *REF: Kandel 1952; Frank et al. 2007a p. 276*

KASABACH METHOD

AP axial oblique projection of the odontoid process, developed many years ago.
  Patient is supine. Rotate the head 45° away from the side being examined. Centre IR 10° ↓ to a point midway between the outer canthus and the EAM. *REF: Kasabach 1939; Ballinger & Frank 1999a p. 391*

KISCH METHOD

Axiolateral projection of femoral head, neck and upper femur.
  Roll the patient towards the affected side. Position leg in lateral position. Angle IR 15–20° ↑ to mid-femoral neck. *REF: Ballinger & Frank 1999a p. 353*

See FRIEDMAN METHOD.

KITE METHODS

Projections to demonstrate clubfoot.

AP and lateral projections of foot at 90° without any attempt to straighten the foot. *REF: Frank et al. 2007a pp. 272–274*

KNUTSSON METHOD

Skyline patella.

Position the patient supine, or seated. Knee flexed. Centre IR to the tibia directed through patellofemoral joint space towards the image receptor placed beyond the apex of the flexed knee so the patella is projected onto it. The degree of IR angle is dependent on the amount of knee flexion but should be 15–20° ↑ from the horizontal. *REF: Merchant et al. 1974*

KOVACS METHOD

Profile image of the lowermost lumbar intervertebral foramen.

The patient lies on the affected side. Rotate the pelvis 30° anteriorly. Centre along a straight line extending from the superior edge of the uppermost iliac crest through the fifth lumbar segment to the inguinal region of the dependent side. Collimate to the foramen of interest. *REF: Kovacs 1950; Ballinger & Frank 1999a pp. 438–439*

KUCHENDORF METHOD

Oblique PA projection of the patella.

Patient is prone; elevate the hip of the affected side and slightly flex the knee so it is parallel with the receptor. Centre IR to the joint space between the patella and the femoral condyles and angle of 30° ↓. *REF: Frank et al. 2007a p. 320*

KURZBAUER METHOD

Axiolateral projection of the sternoclavicular articulation.

Patient lies on the affected side with the arm of that side next to the head. IR is angled 15° ↓ to the sternoclavicular articulation closest to the cassette. *REF: Ballinger & Frank 1999a p. 488*

LAQUERRIERE AND PIERQUIN METHOD (ULNAR GROOVE)

Supero-inferior, PA axial projection of ulnar groove.

Seat patient at the end of table so that the forearm is able to rest flat on the table, hand up, and also parallel to long axis of table. Receptor is under the elbow. Flex the elbow so that the humerus makes an angle of 75° with the forearm. IR is perpendicular to ulnar groove, therefore 15° to long axis of the humerus, at a point just medial to olecranon process. Described but not named in *REF: Frank et al. 2007a p. 157*

LAQUERRIERE AND PIERQUIN METHOD (SCAPULAR SPINE)

Tangential projection of the spine of the scapula.

Patient is supine, rotated so that the scapular is horizontal. CR 45° ↓ through posterosuperior aspect of the shoulder. 35° is sufficient for obese or round-shouldered patients. *REF: Frank et al. 2007a pp. 222–223*

LAUENSTEIN

Routine mediolateral ' frog leg' hip projection demonstrating the acetabulum and proximal femur. *REF: Ballinger & Frank 1999a pp. 344-5; Bontrager 1997 p. 240*

LAUENSTEIN AND HICKEY METHOD

Mediolateral projection of hip with 20–25° angulation ↑ to project the femoral neck free of superimposition by the greater trochanter. *REF: Frank et al. 2007a pp. 356–357*

LAURIN'S METHOD

Tangential projection of patella with 20° flexion to measure the lateral patellofemoral angle with both patellae in the image, as in MERCHANT'S METHOD. *REF: http://www.wheelessonline.com/ortho/axilla_view_of_the_patella; Laurin et al. 1979*

LAWRENCE METHOD (1)

Lateral view of the proximal humerus.

Supine, horizontal beam axial shoulder. Patient is supine with arm abducted 90°. IR directed IS and 15–30° medially depending on degree of abduction to ensure perpendicularity and coverage of the limb on the resultant radiograph. *REF: http.//www. emedicine.com/orthoped/topic464.htm*

LAWRENCE METHOD (2)

Transthoracic lateral humerus.

Patient is in lateral position, raise unaffected arm and rest on head, elevate this shoulder as much as possible to lower affected shoulder. Expose on full inspiration. If patient cannot elevate unaffected shoulder, angle IR 10–15° ↑ to obtain comparable radiograph. This is a grid-based high-dose projection that should be used as a last resort due to the structures along the path of the beam. *REF: Frank et al. 2007a pp. 180–183; Bontrager 1997 p. 163*

LENTINO METHOD

See CARPAL BRIDGE VIEW. *REF: Lentino et al. 1957; Frank et al. 2007a p. 137 fig. 4:96*

LEONARD-GEORGE METHOD

Demonstrates the femoral head and neck.

Patient is supine. A curved cassette is placed on the medial aspect of the leg of interest (between the thighs). Direct the central ray perpendicular to the femoral neck in a lateromedial direction. May not be possible today due to use of curved cassette though it may be possible to place an 18 × 24 cm flat receptor in a similar way. *REF: Ballinger & Frank 1999a p. 350*

LEQUESNE METHOD (FALSE PROFILE VIEW)

View of the posterior rim of acetabulum in profile.

Patient stands with their back against the vertical bucky. Move the unaffected hip forward so that the pelvis makes an angle of 60° with the bucky. IR perpendicular to film through affected hip. Also termed URIST'S METHOD.

LETOURNEL METHOD

AP and PA Iliac wing projections.

AP – (RPO or LPO) from a supine position raise and support the unaffected side 40° to enable the blade of the ilium to fall parallel with the plane of the receptor in the bucky. Centre a vertical IR at the level of the ASIS and collimate to include whole of ilium.

PA – (RAO or LAO) from a prone position elevate the unaffected side 40° so the iliac blade is perpendicular to the image receptor. The patient should use the forearm and bent leg to support. Centre a vertical IR at ASIS level and collimate to include all area.

Described but not named in *REF: Frank et al. 2007a p. 369*

LEWIS METHOD (SESAMOID BONES)

Tangential projection of the sesamoid bones of the first metatarsal.

Patient is prone with toes dorsiflexed against cassette. IR perpendicular and tangential to first metatarsophalangeal joint. *REF: Frank et al. 2007a pp. 252–253*

LEWIS METHOD (THUMB)

Similar to LONG AND RAFERT METHOD.

Position the patient as for AP thumb. IR angled 10–15° proximally along long axis of thumb centring to MCP joint. *REF: Frank et al. 2007a p. 111*

LILIENFELD METHOD (CALCANEUM)

See COALITION VIEW. Demonstrates a calcaneotalar coalition.

Patient standing with the receptor under the long axis of the calcaneum. Angle the IR 45° and direct it through the posterior surface of the flexed ankle to the level of the base of the fifth metatarsal. *REF: Ballinger & Frank 1999a p. 265*

LILIENFELD METHOD (HIP)

A posterolateral projection of the ilium and acetabulum. This is rarely performed now due to the use of CT.

Position the patient prone then raise the unaffected side by 75°. Centre vertical IR at the level of the greater trochanter of the hip in contact with the film. *REF: Ballinger & Frank 1999a p. 356*

See COLONNA METHOD for variation on this projection where patient lies on unaffected side. *REF: Ballinger & Frank 1999a p. 356*

LILIENFELD METHOD (SYMPHYSIS PUBIS)

A superoinferior projection of the pubic and ischial bones and symphysis pubis.

Position as for AP pelvis then raise the body by 45°. Centre IR in the midline at the level of the greater trochanter. This creates a similar result to using the TAYLOR METHOD. *REF: Frank et al. 2007a p. 367; Bontrager & Lampignano 2010 p. 277*

See also STAUNIG METHOD for PA variation. *REF: Ballinger & Frank 1999a – p362*

LINDBÖLM METHOD

AP, LPO or RPO lordotic position for lung apices.

Patient leans back 30+°, centre IR to mid-sternum and collimate to include both apices. *REF: Frank et al. 2007a pp. 534–535*

LONG AND RAFERT METHOD (THUMB)

Position patient as for AP thumb. Angle IR 15° proximally to long axis of thumb centring at CMC joint. *REF: Frank et al. 2007a p. 111*

LOWENSTEIN'S VIEW

AP oblique projection of both hips, particularly to evaluate comparatively for slipped upper femoral epiphysis.

Position the patient supine with the knees flexed and legs abducted so the soles of the feet are in contact. Ensure the femora are matched in their positions relative to the top of the examination table. Centre the IR perpendicular to image receptor at a point 2.5 cm superior to symphysis pubis. *REF: Frank et al. 2007a p. 350; Bontrager & Lampignano 2010 p. 270*

LUNGE POSITION

Weight-bearing lateral foot with ankle flexed.

Patient stands on a block so foot is lateral to the image receptor placed along the medial side of the extremity. Patient leans forwards. Centre horizontal IR to base of third metatarsal.

See SCHUSS POSITION.

MACQUEEN-DELL

Transpharyngeal view of the head of the mandibular condyle.

The image receptor is parallel to the median sagittal plane and centred to the EAM of the affected side. The central ray is angled 5° ↑ and 5° posteriorly towards the condyle to be examined.

MAY METHOD

PA tangential projection of the zygomatic arch.

Position the patient prone or erect PA with the chin raised as far as possible. The head is then rotated 15° away from the side being examined, then tilt the top of the head 15° away from side of interest. IR perpendicular to IOML through the zygomatic arch of interest. *REF: Ballinger & Frank 1999b p. 330*

MERCEDES VIEW

Routine superior-inferior axial shoulder view, or lateral scapula view.

MERCHANT'S METHOD

Tangential view of the patella utilising a cassette-holding device. Patient is supine. Knees flexed 45° over the end of the table. Position femora so that they are parallel to the table top. Strap knees and feet together. Angle the central ray 30° ↓ from the horizontal (30° to femora). Centre midway between patellae. *REF: Frank et al. 2007a pp. 322–323; Bontrager & Lampignano 2010 p. 254; Merchant et al. 1974*

MILLER'S METHOD

Also termed GARTH METHOD.

To demonstrate anterior or posterior dislocation of the shoulder.

Position the patient in AP oblique position. The tube is then angled 45° towards the feet and centred to the glenoid. If the head of the humerus is projected below the glenoid then the dislocation is anterior. If the head of the humerus is projected above the glenoid then the dislocation is posterior. *REF: Bontrager 1997 p.164*

MODIFIED CLEAVES METHOD

Bilateral frog-leg lateral hips, both femora abducted 40–45° from vertical. Centre IR midline, perpendicular to and 2.5 cm above symphysis pubis. *REF: Frank et al. 2007a p. 350; Bontrager & Lampignano 2010 p. 276*

MODIFIED TOWNES PROJECTION

Demonstrates condyloid processes of mandible and temporomandibular fossa.

Position the patient AP without rotation OML perpendicular to film. CR 35° ↓ from OML to pass through at level of TMJs. May be done with patient's mouth open and closed for comparison. *REF: Frank et al. 2007b pp. 376–377; Bontrager & Lampignano 2010 p. 435*

MONDA METHOD

Lateral cervicodorsal junction with patient in lateral recumbent position, 'swimmer's' lateral. Arm closest to image receptor is raised above the head and the humeral head eased anteriorly. The arm furthest from the cassette rests against the patient's side, the humeral head is eased posteriorly and depressed as much as possible. IR 5–15° ↓ to C7–D1 disc space. See also PAWLOW METHOD.

MORTISE VIEW

AP with 15–20° medial rotation of ankle. Intermalleolar line is parallel to film. Centre vertical IR midway between malleoli. *REF: Frank et al. 2007a pp. 290–291; Bontrager & Lampignano 2010 p. 236*

NEER METHOD (SUBSCAPULAR OUTLET TANGENTIAL PROJECTION)

To demonstrate the acromiohumeral space, shoulder impingement or osteophytosis.

Position the patient erect in PA lateral scapular position. Centre IR 10–15° ↓ to superior margin of humeral head. *REF: Frank et al. 2007a p. 194; Bontrager & Lampignano 2010 p. 195*

NORGAARD METHOD (BALL CATCHER'S VIEW)

AP oblique projection of both hands to show small joint erosions in rheumatoid arthritis.

Supination of each hand to an angle of 45° with the fingers cupped as if to catch a ball. Centre midway between the heads of the fifth metacarpals. *MAY* be performed without cupping of fingers. *REF: Frank et al. 2007a pp. 122–123*

OPPENHEIM'S METHOD

Cephaloscapular projection.

X-ray beam passed from superior to inferior across the glenoid face to an image receptor behind the patient, who is leaning forward. Similar projection, tangential view of the scapular spine described but not named. *REF: Frank et al. 2007a pp. 224–225*

Patient is seated with back against table with image receptor behind patient, supported by a sponge making an angle of 45° to the table. IR directed through the anterosuperior aspect of the shoulder at a postero-inferior angle of 45°, i.e. perpendicular to the cassette.

OTTONELLO METHOD

AP cervical spine with moving jaw. Use low mA and long exposure time. *REF: Bontrager & Lampignano 2010 p. 314*

OUTLET VIEW (SHOULDER)

Supraspinatus outlet view. See NEER METHOD (SUBSCAPULAR OUTLET TANGENTIAL PROJECTION).

PAWLOW METHOD

Lateral cervicodorsal junction. Known as swimmer's lateral.

Patient in lateral recumbent position. Arm closest to image receptor raised above the head and the humeral head eased anteriorly. The arm furthest from the cassette rests on the patient's side, the humeral head is eased posteriorly and depressed as much as possible. CR 3–5° to C7–T1 disc space. *REF: Frank et al. 2007a p. 3*

See also MONDA METHOD – same patient position with a 5–15° tube tilt cephalad. *REF: Frank et al. 2007a p. 413.* See also TWINING METHOD – patient erect C4–T3. *REF: Frank et al. 2007a p. 413; Bontrager & Lampignano 2010 p. 311*

PEARSON METHOD

A bilateral AP projection of the acromioclavicular joints.

Both joints taken in one exposure on a wide image receptor, with and without weights. *REF: Frank et al. 2007a pp. 202–203*

Described but not named in *REF: Bontrager & Lampignano 2010 pp. 198–199 (erect and supine methods described)*

PENNAL'S METHOD (TILE'S METHOD)

Trauma views to show the pelvic inlet and outlet.

1 Patient is positioned as for an AP pelvis. Angle the central ray 40° ↓ and centre midway between the ASIS. May also be termed Bridgeman when centring at the level of the greater trochanters. *REF: Frank et al. 2007a p. 368; Bontrager & Lampignano 2010 p. 278*
2 Patient is positioned as for an AP pelvis. Angle the central ray 40° ↑ and centre in the midline 4 cm below the upper border of the symphysis pubis. May be termed Taylor method. *REF: Frank et al. 2007a p. 367; Bontrager & Lampignano 2010 p. 276; Tile et al. 2002 chapter 15*

PENNER

See DUNLAP, SWANSON AND PENNER METHOD. Projection to show the acetabulae in profile.

PIERQUIN METHOD

Projection demonstrates ulnar sulcus obscured due to calcification.

Position the patient seated so that the forearm is rested on the table parallel to its long axis, with hand supinated. The humerus makes angle of 75° to the forearm. IR perpendicular to ulnar sulcus just medial to olecranon process. Described but not named in *REF: Frank et al. 2007a p. 157*

PILLAR VIEWS

AP axial oblique projections of the cervical spine to demonstrate the posterior vertebral arches. Uses right and left head rotations.

Position as for AP cervical spine. Take two exposures, one with the head rotated at 45–50° to the left and one with the head rotated similarly to the right. Angle the vertical central ray 30–40° ↓ and centre the IR just behind the angle of the mandible with the top of the image receptor at the level of the EAM. *REF: Frank et al. 2007a pp. 410–411 (AP axial projections with 20–30° ↓); Frank et al. 2007a p. 412 (axial obliques)*

PIRIE

This is the routine occipitomental 30° sinus view with the mouth open. Described as 'open-mouthed Waters'. *REF: Frank et al. 2007b pp. 400–401; Bontrager 1997 p. 401; Goldman & Cope 1993*

PRAYER POSITION

Lateral calcanei.

The patient's legs abducted and the plantar surfaces of the feet placed together. Centre between the heels to include both heels on the resultant image.

QUESADA METHOD

Projections of the clavicle.

Position the patient prone.

1 Centre to the midpoint of the clavicle at an angle of 15–30° ↓.
2 Alternatively a lordotic position may be adopted with the erect patient using an AP beam 0–15° ↑ IR or similarly the patient may be supine.

A tangential projection of the clavicle is possible with the image receptor resting at the superior surface of the shoulder to make an angle with the table top of 70°. The IR is angled 25–40° from a horizontal start point and tilted ↓ to produce a grazing projection inferosuperiorly of the clavicle. Described but not named in *REF: Frank et al. 2007a pp. 209–211*

RAFERT-LONG METHOD

Scaphoid series PA wrist, extreme ulnar deviation, angle 0, 10, 20 and 30°↑ toward the forearm. The scaphoid is demonstrated with minimal superimposition. *REF: Frank et al. 2007a p. 134*

REVERSE TOWNES

See also HÄÄS METHOD. PA axial skull. *REF: Frank et al. 2007b pp. 322–323; Bontrager & Lampignano 2010 p. 397*

REVERSE WATERS

AP method for facial bones for use on trauma patients. Patient is AP without rotation of head. Centre IR parallel to mentomeatal line and therefore 37° to OML. Centre to bucky and expose to include all facial bones. *REF: Frank et al. 2007b p. 356; Bontrager & Lampignano 2010 p. 622*

ROBERT'S METHOD

See also LONG AND RAFERT METHOD and LEWIS METHOD. True AP thumb. *REF: Frank et al. 2007a pp. 110–111*

Described as modified Robert's method. *REF: Bontrager & Lampignano 2010 p. 145*

ROSENBERG METHOD

PA knees, weight-bearing.

Knees are flexed to place femurs at 45° relative to vertical bucky. Centre IR between a horizontal to 10°↓ to pass through femorotibial joint space. Image is similar to intercondylar knee projection but demonstrates articular surfaces clearly for degenerative changes. *REF: Frank et al. 2007a p. 309; Bontrager & Lampignano 2010 p. 247; Rosenberg et al. 1988*

SANDERSON METHOD

Mediolateral projection of the hip as a trauma or mobile presentation so similar to CLEMENTS NAKAYAMA METHOD.

The image receptor is placed partially under the affected hip and angled parallel to the long axis of the foot. The IR is angled mediolaterally to be perpendicular to long axis of foot, therefore 90° to image receptor. Angulation of the IR 10–20° will better visualise neck and head of femur if grid can also be angled to prevent grid cut-off. *REF: Frank et al. 2007a p. 360; Bontrager & Lampignano 2010 p. 284 (Clements Nakayama)*

SCHNEIDER METHOD

Demonstrates the upper contour of the femoral head.

1 Patient is supine with the femur flexed 60°.
2 Patient is supine with the femur flexed 30°.

Vertical IR centred to the hip joint.

SCHÜLLER

Submento-vertex projection of the skull base.
    Position the patient either in erect seated position or supine with shoulders elevated on a radiolucent mattress. Extend the neck to rest the vertex of the head against the image receptor bucky. Attempt to ensure the OMBL is parallel with the receptor. Centre the IR to the mid-sagittal line in the centre of the skull with angulation if necessary to enable the IR to be perpendicular to the receptor. Collimate to include the whole of the cranium. *REF: Frank et al. 2007b pp. 324–325; Bontrager & Lampignano 2010 p. 396 (variation described for supine patient)*

SCHUSS POSITION

Lateral foot weight-bearing, ankle flexed. Centre IR to base of third metatarsal. Demonstrates longitudinal arch movement when weight-bearing.
    See LUNGE POSITION.

SERENDIPITY (ROCKWOOD) METHOD

View of the sternoclavicular joints for possible dislocation.
    Position the patient supine. Centre IR 40°↑ through manubrium of sternum. A longer SID will be necessary: 150 cm in adults and 115 cm in children. Adjust exposure to account for the

increased distances. An anteriorly or posteriorly dislocated clavicle will be projected above or below the level of correctly enlocated clavicle. *REF: Cope 1993; Bucholz et al. 2010 p. 1248; Long & Rafert 1995 pp. 216–217*

SETTEGAST METHOD

Tangential projection of the patella.

Position the patient supine, prone, lateral or seated. Knee flexed. Centre IR to the tibia directed through patellofemoral joint space towards the image receptor placed beyond the apex of the flexed knee so the patella is projected onto it. The degree of IR angle is dependent on the amount of knee flexion but should be 15–20° ↑ from the horizontal, or plane parallel with the patella in the case of the patient turned laterally. *REF: Frank et al. 2007a pp. 324–325; Bontrager & Lampignano 2010 pp. 255–257*

SKYLINE METACARPAL HEAD

This skyline projection demonstrates vertical impaction fracture in the metacarpal head. Supinate the injured hand, clenching the fist so that the metacarpal head is in profile. Centre vertical IR tangential to MC head, collimnating to include digits of interest. *REF: Eyres & Allen 1993*

SKYLINE PATELLA

Any axial or tangential projection of the patella.

SIMMONS METHOD

To demonstrate congenital talipes equinovarus.

1 AP of both feet with the X-ray tube angled 30° to the hindfoot.
2 AP of each foot with the foot held in the position of fullest correction. The X-ray tube is angled 30° to the hindfoot.
3 Lateral of each foot. The image receptor is placed against the medial aspect of the foot and a horizontal beam is used.

REF: Simmons 1977

STAUNIG METHOD

An inferosuperior projection of the pubic and ischial bones and symphysis pubis.

Position the patient prone. Centre to the symphysis pubis with the central ray angled 35° ↑. *REF: Ballinger & Frank 1999a p. 363*

See also LILIENFELD METHOD for AP variation. *REF: Frank et al. 2007a p. 367*

STECHER METHODS

Projections of the scaphoid.

1 PA wrist position with the image receptor inclined by 20° so that the hand is higher than the wrist. Centre vertical IR to the scaphoid.
2 PA wrist position with the forearm horizontal and the IR angled 20° towards the elbow. Achieves image outcomes similar to projection above, without image receptor inclination.
3 PA wrist position with the fist clenched. This position tends to widen the fracture line.

REF: Stecher 1937; Frank et al. 2007a pp. 132–133; Bontrager & Lampignano 2010 p. 156 (modified version)

STORK METHOD

See FLAMINGO METHOD. Demonstrates subluxation of the symphysis pubis.

Patient is erect, resting pelvis against erect bucky. A horizontal incident ray is centred on the symphysis pubis. Patient has two projections taken with alternate leg raised from the ground to place the symphysis under stress. Collimate to include whole of symphysis pubis.

STRYKER 'NOTCH' METHOD

Demonstrates defects on posterolateral aspect of the humeral head or the Hill-Sachs defect.

Patient is erect or supine with hand on head. Elbow forward, humerus perpendicular to film. Centre IR 10° ↑ towards the coracoid process. *REF: Frank et al. 2007a p. 195*

SUNRISE PATELLA PROJECTION

Axial patella projection to demonstrate patella dislocations.

Position the patient on table with knee flexed 25–30° with and without external rotation of tibia. Centre IR tangential to patella. Can be performed as Settegast, Hughston, inferosuperior either sitting, supine or turned laterally to affected side with a horizontal ray directed along long axis of the table. *REF: Frank et al. 2007a pp. 324–325; Bontrager & Lampignano 2010 pp. 255–256; emedicine.com/sports/topic95htm*

SUPRASPINATUS OUTLET VIEW

See NEER METHOD.

SVEN-JOHANNSON METHOD

Horizontal beam lateral hip as in Danelius-Miller approach.

SWANSON METHOD

See DUNLAP, SWANSON AND PENNER METHOD. Projection to show the acetabula in profile.

SWIMMER'S PROJECTION

Lateral C7–T1.

Patient with hand on head to pull humeral head anterior, other shoulder down and humeral head slightly posterior. Horizontal IR centred to include whole of cervical and upper three thoracic vertebra. Expose on expiration. *REF: Frank et al. 2007a p. 413; Bontrager & Lampignano 2010 p. 311 (as in Twining method)*

TALAR NECK VIEW

AP oblique foot.

Patient lies supine. The knee is flexed so that the sole of the foot is in contact with the image receptor then internally rotate the foot by 15°. Centre IR angled 15° towards the midfoot. Also termed Canale view, Kelly view, Canale and Kelly view. *REF: Archdeacon & Wilbur 2002*

TARRANT METHOD

This method is used to demonstrate the clavicle clear of the ribs. It is particularly useful with patients who cannot assume the lordotic or recumbent positions.

Patient sits with the cassette on the lap. Centre IR 25–35° anterior and inferior to the mid-shaft of the clavicle (i.e. directed from behind the patient). The central ray is at right angles to the longitudinal axis of the clavicle. Due to the path of the IR this method is not recommended for radiation protection reasons unless an alternative is not available. The best alternative is described in *REF: Frank et al. 2007a p. 210* where the patient is prone and an exposure to the receptor in the table bucky is employed. *REF: Tarrant 1950*

TAYLOR METHOD (PELVIS)

An inferosuperior projection of the pubic and ischial rami.

Position as for AP pelvis. Centre IR 5 cm distal to the upper border of the symphysis pubis with a 25° ↑ angulation (♂) or a 40° ↑ angulation (♀). *REF: Frank et al. 2007a p. 367; Bontrager & Lampignano 2010 p. 276*

TEMPLETON AND ZIM METHOD

Supero-inferior carpal tunnel projection.

The forearm is placed at right angles to the image receptor with the hand in contact with the cassette. Direct the IR through the carpal tunnel at an angle of 40° towards the fingers from behind the patient. *REF: Templeton & Zim 1964*

See also GAYNOR-HART METHOD or modified Lentino projection. *REF: Frank et al. 2007a pp. 138–139; Bontrager & Lampignano 2010 p. 158; Frank et al. 2007a p. 137*

TEUFEL METHOD

To show the acetabulum and femoral head margin including the fovea capitis.

Patient is in a 35–40° anterior oblique position. Centre IR 2.5 cm superior to the level of the greater trochanter closest to image receptor with 12° ↑ angulation. *REF: Frank et al. 2007a pp. 362–363; Bontrager & Lampignano 2010 p. 280*

TILE'S METHOD

See PENNAL'S METHOD. Trauma views to show the pelvic inlet and outlet.

TITTERINGTON METHOD

The routine occipitomental 30° projection for faciomaxillary sinuses. Similar to WATERS METHOD with 30° ↓ of the IR.

TOMAS AND PROUBASTA

Trauma projection to demonstrate the radial head.

Forearm supinated in contact with cassette, elbow slightly flexed. IR directed 45° mediolaterally to radial head. *REF: Bucholz & Heckman 2001 p. 941; Tomas & Proubasta 1998*

TOWNES PROJECTION

AP axial skull.

IR 30° ↓ OML line or 37°↓ to IOML, whichever is perpendicular to film. Centre IR at midsagittal plane to pass through 2 cm superior to EAMs. *REF: Frank et al. 2007b pp. 316–321; Bontrager & Lampignano 2010 p. 392*

TUBEROSITY VIEW

View of the elbow.

With the elbow AP angle IR 20° towards the olecranon. Various degrees of rotation are used to bring the tuberosity to advantage.

TWINING METHOD

Lateral C4–T3 with patient in erect position, similar to SWIMMER'S PROJECTION. *REF: Frank et al. 2007a p. 413; Bontrager & Lampignano 2010 p. 311 (as in Twining method)*

URIST'S METHOD

View of the acetabular rim in profile.

Patient is supine, injured side elevated 60°. Similar in approach to a further rotated Judet projection. See also LEQUESNE

METHOD. *REF: Frank et al. 2007a pp. 364–366; Bontrager 1997 p. 237*

VEIHWEGER METHOD

Ulnar groove projection.

Position the patient seated with back to table, arm extended from the shoulder to enable the elbow to flex to approx 35° and rest on the image receptor that is on the table top. Centre IR through ulnar groove so it is perpendicular to image receptor.

Described but not named. *REF: Clark 1979 p. 37*

WALLACE-HELLIER PROJECTION

View of the shoulder to generate axiolateral of glenohumeral joint and subacromial space. Has value for dislocation of the shoulder for some trauma presentations. May also be termed the Nottingham view.

The patient sits with their back to the table and the affected shoulder is turned towards the table so that the blade of the scapula is parallel with the table side. Image receptor rests on table top and vertical IR is angled 30° towards the anterior aspect of the shoulder. Centre to the shoulder joint. A larger source to image distance should be considered to counter magnification; adjust exposure from AP shoulder to suit increased distances employed. *REF: Wallace & Hellier 1983*

WATERS METHOD

The routine occipitomental view of the sinuses.

Position the patient PA to erect bucky with OML 37° to image receptor. Midsagittal plane is perpendicular to the midline of erect bucky. Centre IR perpendicular to image receptor so that it exits at the acanthion. Ask patient to drop lower jaw to allow sphenoidal sinuses to be demonstrated. *REF: Frank et al. 2007b p. 352; Bontrager & Lampignano 2010 p. 420*

WEST POINT SHOULDER (WEST POINT AXILLARY LATERAL)

To demonstrate chronic shoulder instability, anterior inferior glenoid abnormalities and Hill-Sachs lesions.

Named Radiography Projections

Patient is prone with shoulder raised on a pad and head turned away from affected side. Abduct arm so that the forearm of the affected shoulder lies over the side of the table. Support image receptor against superior aspect of shoulder. Centre to the axilla and angle IR 25° downward from the horizontal and 25° medially. *REF: Frank et al. 2007a pp. 184–185*

WILLIAMS METHOD

Projection to demonstrate the costovertebral and costotransverse joints.

Patient is supine. Angle the IR 20° ↑ and centre to T6. Collimate to include the whole of the thoracic spine to show all the above joints. Described but not named in *REF: Frank et al. 2007a pp. 496–497*

Y VIEW

PA oblique or lateral scapula.

IR is perpendicular to film through scapulohumeral joint. By placing the arm in multiple positions on the affected side differing facets of the scapula will be shown.

Anterior oblique: shows scapula spine and coracoid process. *REF: Bontrager & Lampignano 2010 p. 194*

Prone or erect 45–60° RAO or LAO:

1 Flex elbow to rest forearm on back to show acromion and coracoid. *REF: Frank et al. 2007a pp. 214–215*
2 Extend forearm and rest on head to show scapular body.
3 Lorenz version has patient lying on affected side with upper arm at right angles to the body and hand resting by the head. Lilienfeld describes a similar position but with the arm extended upwards obliquely so the elbow can be flexed to allow the hand to rest on the head. Both methods deliver a slightly oblique projection of the scapula. *REF: Frank et al. 2007a pp. 216–217*

Neer method: patient in same position but IR is angled 15° ↓ to scapulohumeral joint.

ZANCA'S METHOD

As for the routine view of the acromioclavicular joint but with a 10–15° ↑ tilt of the IR. See ALEXANDER METHOD. *REF: Frank et al. 2007a pp. 204–205; Bucholz & Heckman 2001 p. 1219*

ZANELLI METHOD

Projection to demonstrate the TMJs in the open and closed positions.

Patient is lateral with the head 30° away from the vertical, i.e. top of head against the image receptor. Centre 2.5 cm anterior to the EAM and expose with mouth open and then closed to show articulation. This is similar to the axiolateral oblique described in *REF: Frank et al. 2007b pp. 372–374*

ZITER'S VIEW

Scaphoid view.

Wrist PA with ulnar deviation. Angle the tube 25° ↑ towards the elbow and centre between the styloid processes. *REF: Wallace & Hellier 1983*

See STECHER METHODS. *REF: Stecher 1937; Frank et al. 2007a pp. 132–133; Bontrager & Lampignano 2010 p. 156 (modified version)*

References

Anderson I.F., Read J.W. and Steinweg J. (1998) *Atlas of Imaging in Sports Medicine*. McGraw Hill, Sydney, London.

Archdeacon M. and Wilbur R. (2002) Fractures of the talar neck. *Orthopedic Clinics of North America* 33(1): 248–262.

Ballinger P.W. and Frank E.D. (1999a) *Merrill's Atlas of Radiographic Positioning and Radiologic Procedures* 9th Ed Vol 1. Mosby/Elsevier, St Louis, MO.

Ballinger P.W. and Frank E.D. (1999b) *Merrill's Atlas of Radiographic Positioning and Radiologic Procedures* 9th Ed Vol 2. Mosby/Elsevier, St Louis, MO.

Bontrager K.L. (1997) *Textbook of Radiographic Positioning and Related Anatomy* 4th Ed. Mosby/Elsevier, St Louis, MO.

Bontrager K.L. and Lampignano J.P. (2010) *Textbook of Radiographic Positioning and Related Anatomy* 7th Edn. Mosby/Elsevier, St Louis, MO.

Bucholz R.W. and Heckman J.D. (2001) *Rockwood & Greens Fractures in Adults* 5th Ed. Lippincott Williams & Wilkins, Philadelphia, PA.

Bucholz R.W., Court-Brown C.C., Heckman J.D. and Tornetta P. III (2010) *Rockwood & Greens Fractures in Adults* 7th Ed. Lippincott Williams & Wilkins, Philadelphia, PA.

Carver E. and Carver B. (2006) *Medical Imaging: Techniques, Reflection and Evaluation*. Churchill Livingstone/Elsevier, Edinburgh.

Clark K. (1979) *Clark's Positioning in Radiography* 10th Ed. Heinemann Medical Books Ltd, London.

Conway W.F., Destout J.M., Gilula L.A. et al. (1985) The carpal boss: an overview of radiographic evaluation. *Radiology* 156: 29–31.

Cope R. (1993) Dislocations of the sternoclavicular joints. *Skeletal Radiology* 22: 233–238.

Coyle G.F. (1980) Unit 7, Special angled views of joints: elbow, knee, ankle. In: *Radiographing Immobile Trauma Patients*. Multi-Media Publishing, Inc., Denver, CO.

Dye M.T. (2000) Metacarpal Fractures. *http://emedicine.com/sports/topic95htm*

Eyres K.S. and Allen T.R. (1993) Skyline view of the metacarpal head in the assessment of human fight-bite injuries. *Journal of Hand Surgery* 18B: 43–44.

Fisk, C. (1965) Adaptation of the technique for radiography of the bicipital groove. *Radiologic Technology* 37: 47–50.

Frank E.D., Long B.W. and Smith B.J. (Eds) (2007a) *Merrill's Atlas of Radiographic Positioning and Procedures* 11th Ed, Vol 1. Mosby/Elsevier, St Louis, MO.

Frank E.D., Long B.W. and Smith B.J. (Eds) (2007b) *Merrill's Atlas of Radiographic Positioning and Procedures* 11th Ed, Vol 2. Mosby/Elsevier, St Louis, MO.

Goldman M. and Cope D. (1993) *A Radiographic Index* 8th Ed reprinted. Butterworth Heinemann, Oxford.

Johnson C.R. (1932) A new method for roentgenographic examination of the upper end of the femur. *Journal of Bone and Joint Surgery* 30: 859–866.

Kandel B. (1952) The suproplantar projection in the congenital clubfoot of the infant, *Acta Orthopaedica Scandinavica* 22: 161–173.

Kasabach H.H. (1939) A roentgenographic method for the study of the second cervical vertebrae. *AJR American Journal of Roentgenology* 42: 782–785.

Kovacs, A. (1950) X-ray examination of the exit of the lowermost lumbar root. *Radiologia Clinica* 19: 6–13.

Laurin C, Dussalut R and Levesque H.P. (1979) The tangential X-ray investigation of the patello-femoral joint. *Clinical Orthopaedics & Related Research* 144: 16–26.

Lentino W., Lubetsky H.W., Jacobson H.G. et al. (1957) The carpal bridge view. *Journal of Bone and Joint Surgery* 39A: 88–90.

Long B.W. and Rafert J.A. (1995) *Orthopaedic Radiography*. WB Saunders, Philadelphia, PA.

Merchant A.C., Mercer R.L., Jacobsen R.H. and Cool C.R. (1974) Roentgenographic analysis of patellofemoral congruence. *Journal of Bone and Joint Surgery* 56A(7): 1391–1396.

Rockwood C.A., Green D.P., Bucholz R.W. and Heckman J.D. (1996) *Rockwood & Green's Fractures in Adults* 4th Ed. Lippincott Williams & Wilkins, Philadelphia, PA.

Rosenberg T.D., Paulos L.E., Parker RD, Coward D.B. and Scott S.M. (1988) The forty-five degree posteroanterior flexion weight-bearing radiograph of the knee. *Journal of Bone and Joint Surgery* 70A: 1479–1483.

Simmons G.W. (1977) Analytical radiographs of club foot. *Journal of Bone and Joint Surgery* 59B(4): 485–489.

Skripkus J.U. and Gentili A (2006) Radiographic evaluation. In Davies M. et al. *Imaging of the Hip and Bony Pelvis: Techniques and Applications.* Springer, Berlin.

Stecher W.R. (1937) Roentgenography of the carpal navicular bone. *AJR American Journal of Roentgenology* 37:704–705.

Tarrant R.M. (1950) The axial view of the clavicle. *X-ray Technician* 21: 358–359.

Templeton A.W. and Zim I.D. (1964) The carpal tunnel view. *Missouri Medicine* 61: 443–444.

Tile M., Kellam J. and Helfet D. (2002) *Fractures of the Pelvis and Acetabulum* 3rd Ed. Lippincott Williams & Wilkins, Philadelphia, London.

Tomas F.J. and Proubasta I.D. (1998) Modified radial head capitellum projection in elbow trauma. *British Journal of Radiology* 71(841): 74–75.

Wallace H.A. and Hellier M. (1983) Improving radiographs of the injured shoulder. *Radiography* 49: 229–233.

Wheeless' Textbook of Orthopaedics (updated daily) *http://www.wheelessonline.com*

Chapter 5

Procedures Using Contrast Agents +/– Fluoroscopy

Changing modalities over recent history has resulted in the reduction of many fluoroscopically directed examinations. However, some simple rules apply to all the procedures that can be directed to your patient. This section will review the following procedures that remain relatively common:

- Barium swallow
- Barium meal
- Barium followthrough
- Barium enema
- Micturating cystourethrogram
- Cystogram
- Intravenous urogram or pyelogram (IVU/IVP)
- T-tube cholangiogram (fairly uncommon)
- Nephrostogram
- Fistulogram
- Sinugram/sinogram
- Hysterosalpingogram

Each of these requires an explanation to the patient (some needing signed consent) and appropriate preparation to ensure a safe and diagnostic (or even therapeutic) procedure result. Some situations will require alterations to the procedure and consideration of the impact a procedure may have on subsequent investigations. A list of equipment used, possible complications and contraindications is provided.

Index of Medical Imaging, First Edition. Jonathan McConnell.
© 2011 Blackwell Publishing Ltd. Published 2011 by Blackwell Publishing Ltd.

Explanation to the patient

Procedure	Explanation
Barium swallow/meal and followthrough	Drink barium – describe taste Bubble maker – don't burp up the gas (barium meal) Swallow when told to (drink all barium over a short time frame at start of examination) Rolling around for pictures Followthrough – several pictures over several hours, don't eat or drink until finished, timing different for each person Aftercare – remember to hydrate, constipation may need laxatives to ease
Barium enema	What we are doing – many patients think they are just here for an X-ray Check the bowel preparation went OK – take a control film Tube into rectum with balloon on end – will feel like they must go to the toilet Do NOT force out balloon – may cause prolapse Tell them the qualification of who is catheterising Fluid in then out, followed by air – will feel like cramps – don't try to 'expel' the air Lots of rolling around over 20 minutes or so Obtain consent Explain aftercare which is similar to barium meals, etc.
Micturating cystourethrogram and cystogram	Reason for doing this – draw diagram Tell them about the urethral catheter and qualification of who is catheterising Get consent from patient/carer Question if urinary tract infection is present May be uncomfortable – adults cope; child will probably cry, as may be held down Local anaesthetic lubricating jelly used – numb feeling MCU requires patient to 'wet the bed' – child may be 'toilet trained' Tell them we have facility for patient to wash after the examination due to sticky contrast media

Using Contrast Agents +/– Fluoroscopy

Procedure	Explanation
Intravenous urogram or pyelogram (IVU/IVP)	Why we are doing this – how does it work: fluid is filtered by kidney, shows up in urine, shows how kidneys, ureters and bladder are working and their gross anatomy. Several pictures taken X-ray tube may swing over head (tomography), but can't hit them Compression device may be used – question to see if this is contraindicated Urinate before and during examination Must tell us if they are feeling 'funny' or having chest pain or trouble breathing Tell them normal responses – may feel hot, nausea – will go away fairly quickly Question other medications, diseases for potential renal or hepatic complications
T-Tube cholangiogram (fairly uncommon), nephrostogram, fistulogram and sinugram/ sinogram	Why we are doing this – stones? Size of a sinus, fistula? Stenosis of AV fistula for dialysis? Leaks post surgery? Catheter cleaned, fluid (contrast) injected through catheter, pictures taken May require patient to roll around Catheter or needle may be inserted if not present Can get messy if contrast spills out of wound or puncture site May hurt due to pressure May aspirate pus if present, which can have a foul smell
Hysterosalpingogram	Why we are doing this and what we hope to show Reassure there will be minimal staff in room – PRIVACY Tell her qualifications of person performing examination Invasive/sensitive procedure – get consent Reassure minimal radiation dose Similar to internal examination, pap smear – but longer May be cramping Tell her there are clean-up facilities available

Preparation of the patient

Using Contrast Agents +/– Fluoroscopy

Procedure	Preparation
Barium swallow/meal and followthrough	Fast for 12 hours – good to do the examination in the morning, so only breakfast is missed, especially diabetic patient – clean stomach, less likely to vomit Diabetic patient may require meal at end Babies to be fasted for 2 hours No smoking or chewing gum for 6 hours – can increase gastric juices to affect images Warn they may need someone to drive them home, as Buscopan may affect eyesight – check patients for glaucoma as will need glucagon for antispasmodic
Barium enema	Routine cases require full bowel cleansing Indicate need to decrease faecal loading, avoid food that is hard to digest or produces excess gas – can all give confusing results in images Preparation kit (bisacodyl, e.g. Dulcolax) – some preparations require drinking of fluid volumes, others use a tablet preparation. All purge the bowel Fast for 12 hours – a cleansing enema prior may be required Postoperative cases when checking for leaks or fistulae often get no preparation Have replacement stoma bag available, if necessary
Micturating cystourethrogram and cystogram	Some patients demand/require sedation – book in a bed for 4-hour observation after sedation Empty bladder before examination – it can be emptied via the catheter at start of examination Ultrasound may be carried out immediately prior if requested
Intravenous urogram or pyelogram (IVU/IVP)	Fast for 12 hours – patient may have water up to 2 hours prior Bowel preparation may be used though not always required Empty bowels and bladder Check urea and creatinine, if available. Must do if patient in renal failure or on biguanides (metformin-related diabetes control drugs) Ensure patient is well hydrated Check for allergies/sensitivities – may need prophylactic steroids Check for asthma, heart disease, high blood pressure as are contrast media contraindications
T-Tube cholangiogram (fairly uncommon), nephrostogram, fistulogram and sinugram/sinogram	Check contrast allergies/sensitivities Possibly use ultrasound for Arterio-Venous (AV) fistula in arm first before progressing to contrast-based examination
Hysterosalpingogram	Check when last menstrual period started and not currently menstruating Check beta-hCG if possibility of pregnancy Time appointment for examination to occur approximately 10 days following the onset of menstruation May require sedation Recommend someone is available to drive patient home when appointment being booked or information given to patient

Alterations to preparation

Procedure	Preparation
Barium swallow/meal and followthrough	Schedule diabetics for first appointment Alter fasting times for children/infants Should examination be performed if risk of pregnancy
Barium enema	Schedule diabetics early in the day Fit in with transport arrangements for elderly Postpone if pregnant unless clinical urgency overrules Employ minimal bowel preparation (cathartics) for ulcerative colitis, diverticulitis Consideration for enlarged colon Colostomies, ileostomies may require washout on arrival
Micturating cystourethrogram and cystogram	Possible sedation If urinary tract infection – postpone examination Pregnancy – ? postpone
Intravenous urogram or pyelogram (IVU/IVP)	Find out baby's or child's weight to adjust dose of contrast medium Diabetics – first appointment so food may be provided after and reduces hypoglycaemic response Pregnancy – ? postpone Renal impairment, renal failure – check urea and creatinine – remember diabetes and metformin use with intravenous iodinated contrast media may cause acute renal failure if not allowed for Hepatitis, cirrhosis – check bilirubin level (indicator of liver function, therefore likely success of examination)
T-Tube cholangiogram (fairly uncommon), nephrostogram, fistulogram and sinugram/ sinogram	None
Hysterosalpingogram	None

Effects of other medication on the procedures

Procedure	Preparation
Barium swallow/meal and followthrough	Antacids may show up as they do not always dissolve Buscopan will affect a follow through examination as slows the progress Recent CT abdomen – residual contrast will occlude areas of interest esp. if dilute barium solution used Recent barium study – residual contrast will occlude areas of interest
Barium enema	Recent CT abdomen – residual contrast will occlude areas of interest Recent barium study – residual contrast will occlude areas of interest Antacids may show up as they do not always dissolve
Micturating cystourethrogram and cystogram	Recent contrast study may occlude areas of interest General anaesthetic will prevent voluntary micturition
Intravenous urogram or pyelogram (IVU/IVP)	Metformin may affect kidney function or even cause acute renal failure or lactic acidosis (potentially fatal) when contrast is used Recent contrast study may occlude areas of interest Antacids may show up as they do not always dissolve Diuretics, e.g. furosemide (Lasix), may dilute contrast agent thus reducing image contrast
T-Tube cholangiogram (fairly uncommon)	Previous contrast study may occlude areas of interest Antacids may show up as they do not always dissolve
Nephrostogram, fistulogram and sinugram/ sinogram	Recent contrast examination may occlude areas of interest
Hysterosalpingogram	None

Effects of procedures on subsequent examinations

Procedure	Preparation
Barium swallow/meal and followthrough	Need to plan diagnostic tests as will affect timing of other examinations, both before and afterwards as residual contrast will impact Possible constipation – increase drinking after procedure or use laxatives Possible aspiration or leak thus requiring further intervention – other imaging may be affected by leaked or aspirated contrast
Barium enema	Plan the sequence of diagnostic tests as will affect timing of other examinations, both before and afterwards as residual contrast will impact Possible perforation of bowel (following diverticulitis, radiation colitis, ulcerative colitis) Possible constipation, especially in enlarged bowel Possible hypervolaemia (increase in intravascular fluid) – excess water absorbed by enlarged bowel, e.g. Hirschsprung's disease (congenital megacolon)
Micturating cystourethrogram and cystogram	Other contrast examinations residual contrast may occlude areas of imaging Introduce infection – urinary tract infection, cystitis Possible rupture of urethra or bladder
Intravenous urogram or pyelogram (IVU/IVP)	Previous contrast examinations may impact on regional function or occlude for IVU Iodine injected will ruin thyroid uptake examinations (nuclear medicine) for up to 3 months Iodinated contrast will skew results for Bilirubin and other blood tests Possibility of overdose when several examinations with iodinated media done in 24 hours may result in acute renal failure
T-Tube cholangiogram (fairly uncommon), nephrostogram, fistulogram and sinugram/sinogram	Previous contrast examinations may occlude area for imaging As for IVP Possibility of introducing or spreading infections
Hysterosalpingogram	Previous contrast examinations may occlude area being imaged Possibility of affecting embryo or introducing or spreading infection Possibility of embolus via lymphatics if oily media used for examination

Typical equipment used for procedures

Procedure	Preparation
Barium swallow/meal and followthrough	Cup, straw, vomit bowl, tissues Contrast media, mixed as appropriate Other drugs, e.g. Buscopan/glucagon, emergency drugs, negative media (gas producing) Tourniquet, needles, syringes, swabs Pillow, blanket Reading material for followthrough – may take several hours Organise meal for diabetics if necessary post examination
Barium enema	Enema bag, enema tip, inflation device for tip, air introducer for double contrast Lubricant jelly, tissues, gloves Contrast media, mixed as appropriate Other drugs, e.g. Buscopan/glucagon, emergency drugs Tourniquet, needles, syringes, swabs Pillow, blanket Organise meal for diabetics if necessary Commode if necessary, or bedpan Washing up supplies for patient Imaging equipment prepared and easily available to speed examination
Micturating cystourethrogram and cystogram	*Sterile supplies (top shelf):* Catheters, anaesthetic jelly, cleansing solution, sterile tray, gloves, gown, drapes *Nonsterile supplies (bottom shelf):* Sticky tape, contrast, giving set, specimen jar for urine sample *Other:* Side marker, spot light, lead shielding for parent, lead shielding for nurse/radiographer
Intravenous urogram or pyelogram (IVU/IVP)	*Sterile:* IV needle, syringes, syringe filling cannula, dressing pack *Nonsterile:* Contrast, tourniquet, sticky tape, band-aid, emergency drugs *Other:* Compression device (IVU), side marker, positioning/immobilisation sponge, tomographic device, duress button (for patient to raise attention)
T-Tube cholangiogram (fairly uncommon), nephrostogram, fistulogram and sinugram/sinogram	*Sterile:* Syringes, dressing pack, drapes, gloves, connector, needle, syringe filling cannula *Nonsterile:* Antiseptic solution, contrast, saline or water for injection, clamps for tube, replacement collection bag *Other:* Side marker
Hysterosalpingogram	*Sterile:* Tray, speculum, suction device and introducer, syringes, gloves, drapes, gown, syringe filling cannula *Nonsterile:* Antiseptic cream or lotion, contrast, vacuum device *Other:* Side marker, spot light, sanitary pad

Suggested contrast media and doses

Procedure	Preparation
Barium swallow/meal and followthrough	Swallow: barium, e.g. Polibar diluted with water. 1 cup Swallow: gastrografin, GastroView (both ionic). Full strength Swallow: nonionic iodinated water-soluble. 350 mg/mL Meal: as for swallows Meal: also negative contrast to produce double contrast, e.g. medifizz. Consider bubble breaker to ensure good image quality Followthrough: gastrografin, GastroView. Full strength. 240 mL Followthrough: add Entero Vu as per instructions Followthrough: barium, as for meal, 3 cups
Barium enema	Barium: as per manufacturer instructions. Mix up to 1 litre GastroView, gastrografin: full strength, 500 to 1000 mL Nonionic, water-soluble media: 350 mg/mL, 500 to 1000 mL
Micturating cystourethrogram and cystogram	Urografin (ionic): 33% (180 mg/mL), up to 250 mL Possibly nonionic alternative contrast media
Intravenous urogram or pyelogram (IVU/IVP)	IVP: nonionic, water-soluble iodinated media, e.g. Omnipaque 350 mg/mL. Often 50 mL used
T-Tube cholangiogram (fairly uncommon), nephrostogram, fistulogram and sinugram/sinogram	Nonionic, e.g. Omnipaque 180 to 300 mg/mL. Dose as necessary Too dense may obscure stones Take special care not to inject bubbles, as they can mimic stones
Hysterosalpingogram	Water-soluble media: e.g. Omnipaque 180 or 300 mg/mL Mucosal coating not as good as iodised oils. Iodised oils not used, due to possibility of embolus. Also, flow through fallopian tubes could be slow, requiring 24-hour film

Using Contrast Agents +/– Fluoroscopy

Contraindications and procedural precautions

Using Contrast Agents +/– Fluoroscopy

Procedure	Preparation
Barium swallow/meal and followthrough	If chance of aspiration, barium is safer (inert – gastrografin (GastroView) hygroscopic and will draw fluid into the alveolar tissues to generate pneumonitis) Tracheo-oesophageal fistula, barium is safer as above If rupture (oesophagus, stomach) is suspected, barium must not be used – consider diluted nonionic contrast media, e.g. Omnipaque Barium absorbs water, and so can solidify if not enough fluid is taken after examination. Should not be used if there is a high chance of faecal impaction Iodinated contrast media can cause serious dehydration Barium gives better contrast than iodinated media
Barium enema	Enlarged colon – greater surface area to absorb water, leading to barium impaction – use iodinated media. Also absorption can lead to hypervolaemia (important if patient has congestive heart failure) Potential perforation: do NOT use barium – barium peritonitis is likely afterwards
Micturating cystourethrogram and cystogram	Chance of infection
Intravenous urogram or pyelogram (IVU/IVP)	Allergic reaction Assess history before injection Asthma, etc. – prophylactic steroids, e.g. acetylcysteine, may be used Patient must be well hydrated Check vital signs to compare post reaction Not for anuria, thyrotoxicosis, decreased cardiac insufficiency
T-Tube cholangiogram (fairly uncommon), nephrostogram, fistulogram and sinugram/sinogram	Infections and known contrast allergies
Hysterosalpingogram	Infections and known contrast allergies Cannot be performed during or within 5 days of the end of a menstrual cycle

And remember, the role of the radiographer if a nurse is not present (beyond imaging equipment control) is to:

- Explain the procedure
- Check the patient's identity
- Check patient preparation has been successful
- Mix or prepare contrast media, and have other drugs available, e.g. Buscopan, negative contrast, emergency drugs
- Have all accessory equipment available
- Assist radiologist, e.g. positioning patient
- Ensure a safe procedural environment
- Ensure patient care and monitor patient as procedure progresses
- Provide support and encouragement during procedure
- Provide aftercare – cleaning patient, checking welfare
- Clean room and trolley and suction/oxygen if used

Chapter 6

Mobile Radiography and Fluoroscopy

Mobile radiography encompasses work performed on the ward, possibly in the resuscitation room if specialised equipment is not housed there, and using a mobile image intensification system in the operating theatre. The equipment being used is usually not as powerful as plant housed in a typical radiography examination room; however, careful adjustment of exposure factors and development of techniques that minimise exposure can all be applied to procedures performed away from the radiology department.

Radiation protection

Radiation protection techniques should be carefully and consistently applied during these examinations. It is normal for the controlled area around the equipment to be 2 metres in any direction from the source. This can be difficult to achieve for some examinations to be performed on the ward, whereby the direction of the central ray can impact upon other patients or staff (and the public) close by. In these situations, first establish whether it is feasible for the patient to be brought on a bed to the department for the procedure. If this is not possible then, if urgency permits, try to perform the examination at a time when there will be the least number of people in the vicinity of the radiation source. If a problem still exists it may be possible to ask for other patients, visitors and staff to be moved away during the exposure; furthermore, try to direct any central ray away from populated areas. Careful planning is therefore the name of the game.

Index of Medical Imaging, First Edition. Jonathan McConnell.
© 2011 Blackwell Publishing Ltd. Published 2011 by Blackwell Publishing Ltd.

Staff who cannot move away from the radiation source, i.e. the radiographer, operating theatre staff and any personnel such as neonatal nurses who are required to be with the patient during the exposure, should all wear protective lead rubber aprons. Where scattered radiation is generated by a beam of under 100 kVp, a 0.25 mm lead equivalent apron is acceptable. Most staff will be provided with aprons able to resist scatter from a source of 150 kVp thus making the lead rubber 0.35 mm lead equivalent. Especially in the operating theatre where longer exposures may be required, staff should be provided with a thyroid collar and lead glasses, and for the surgeon a choice of thin lead rubber gloves to wear under other sterile gloves should the hands be at risk of entering the area of irradiation.

Techniques

The common examinations performed on the ward include:

- AP chest – semi-erect or supine
- AP supine abdomen
- AP pelvis +/– lateral hip
- Orthopaedic radiography of limbs

For chest images, the key to obtaining good results is achieving an image that is close to erect if possible or, if the patient is supine, using a long source-to-image distance to enable all body parts to be included and to overcome issues linked with magnification and the supine position of the chest radiograph.

To achieve a good erect position, either the back of the patient's bed may be used as direct support, or the moving headrest can be positioned at 45° relative to the mattress with a large foam sponge between. The image receptor is sandwiched between sponge and patient so that a 90° position is possible without moving the patient backwards, thus avoiding any risks to patient due to movement. For a supine image extend the arm of the mobile equipment as far as possible. Place the receptor under the patient, remembering to support the head so a lordotic end position does not result, and centre to the sternal angle. If possible, lower the bed further to increase the source-to-image distance.

Supine abdominal and pelvic examinations are more difficult to achieve due to the need to place the image receptor beneath the patient. Drawer-type devices for the patient to lie on have been developed. This allows easy insertion of the receptor plus grid beneath the patient and enables the surface to be straightened as it is larger than the cassette and can therefore be wedged to achieve a flat aspect, minimising grid cut-off issues. This system also elevates the patient from the mattress, thus enabling clear horizontal ray lateral techniques to be used (central ray direction relative to others in clinical area) or allows a lateral decubitus to be possible. Whichever technique is employed, these examinations are very uncomfortable for the patient and should be performed quickly to minimise pain.

Exposure factors may have to be changed to generate a beam with sufficient power to provide image information. Usually this means a higher kV technique to allow a lower mAs value to be used. Although this will alter the relative image contrast, it will enable the exposure to occur within the power capabilities of the mobile unit and reduce the length of time over which the exposure needs to be delivered, thus reducing the potential for movement unsharpness.

In situations where the patient is infectious or needs to be barrier nursed to prevent infection reaching them, a two-radiographer team approach is adopted. Where the patient is infectious the patient is barrier nursed. Here the radiographer working in the room is the 'dirty' radiographer as they have to deal with the infectious elements of the examination. This person will wear protective equipment that is deposited in sealed bags after use to prevent infection escape prior to the clothing being incinerated after use. Image receptors are covered to prevent transmission outside the patient's room, and the cassette will be cleaned after it is passed out of the room to the receiving 'clean' radiographer. The mobile unit is driven 'X-ray tube first' into the area to minimise the chances of cross-infection. This too is cleaned after the examination. Reverse barrier nursing describes the opposite situation whereby the patient is at great risk of contracting infections due to their immunocompromised status. Here the radiographer working with the patient enters the room (possibly via an anteroom) where full protective garb is applied, i.e. gown, cap, mask, gloves and overshoes, much as in the operating theatre. The image receptor is cleaned and covered by a protective sheath (e.g. pillow case or sterile drape) if needed and used for the examination. The X-ray unit is again cleaned prior to entry into the room and cassettes are passed out to the 'dirty' team member as the machine is reversed out of the room. Again disposable clothing is discarded, this time away from the patient, to minimise the chances of exposure to infection. X-ray equipment is cleaned down before removal from the ward.

Operating theatre situation

Mobile radiographic examinations may be performed using the type of machine seen in ward action or by a mobile fluoroscopy C-arm/image intensifier. Rules already discussed for work in the ward apply in the operating theatre, plus there is a need to ensure that equipment is kept extremely clean due to the potential for cross-infection. Ideally, dedicated equipment is available to the operating suite; however, this is not always possible so good cleaning protocols should be adopted. A sticky pad, over which the equipment is driven on entry to the operating suite, will remove most foreign bodies. Entry to the suite for staff is then via changing rooms so a clean side to the procedure is maintained, and equipment may be swabbed to prepare for use in the theatre. Even if the equipment is kept in the operating suite, movement between theatres requires good cleaning practices.

Those working in the operating theatre will be expected to wear theatre footwear if available (if not, shoe coverings should be applied). Theatre clothing should be changed into with cap and mask used. Sterile gowns and gloves are used by those closely associated with the operating area that must remain sterile.

Modern fluoroscopy systems are able to deliver many imaging menus that will reduce radiation dose to patient and staff. One key point to remember is that if the C-arm system is used with the X-ray tube above the operating site, the radiation dose to the head and upper body of personnel close by is greatly increased. Use of the image intensifier side of the C-arm close to the patient, with the X-ray tube below, minimises dose; by ensuring the receptor is adjacent to the patient, image quality is improved. Keeping the surgical field clean is a potential problem as it would be easy to desterilise the surgeon or patient. Poor technique in cleaning the equipment has been known to result in foreign bodies dropping onto the surgical field – not good for all concerned!

Use of fluoroscopy during hip fracture pinning or to provide guidance during hip replacement surgery requires a specialised technique. The patient is placed on the operating table with legs in a support fastened through a boot. The injured side or side being operated on is placed under traction and fluoroscopy is used to guide the reduction. The uninjured leg is positioned to enable sufficient space for the C-arm unit to be driven in with the intensifier side over the hip. The unit itself is at 90° to the femoral neck so C-arm rotation allows the X-ray tube side to move to generate a lateral beam pointing from opposite the patient's elbow level towards the image intensifier, which is placed close to the femoral neck for image quality. For surgery a large polythene drape is fixed to the operating site and creates a screen between the surgeon and the image intensifier. As the surgeon needs alternative views, the plastic screen maintains a clean operating environment while the C-arm remains draped by the sterile sheet, rotating through 90° for frontal/lateral projections as required.

Where the above system cannot be adopted, elasticated plastic sterile drapes have been created to fix over the C-arm, thus separating it from the operating field. This allows, where possible, close approximation of the intensifier head to the body part without risk of desterilisation of the field.

Unfortunately, the radiographer is frequently called to the operating theatre at a time when setting up of the operating field has been completed; in this situation it may be impossible to achieve the best position (for radiation protection) for fluoroscopy and to minimise radiation dose. This can be improved by using digital pulse sequences and last-image-hold image demonstration techniques so that long-time fluoroscopy (needed for dynamic procedures but which can also be performed using pulse techniques to reduce dose) is avoided. Foot switches are useful to enable operators to work at some distance from equipment that is prepared for use in the procedure when several exposures are needed across time. Good radiation practice would favour this; unfortunately, demands by surgeons to give the foot switch to them may lead to arguments due to overdosing of patients (and staff) because the image intensifier was used too often. In this regrettable situation, image updating appears to be the prime concern rather than radiation protection for all.

Some specialised software functions are available on more modern mobile fluoroscopy units. Today, dual-monitor viewing is the standard whereby previously captured images can be compared against updated ones. Dual monitors also allow previous images to be called back from a store for comparison. Road mapping and subtraction techniques are also used on new equipment. This has made possible vascular procedures in the operating theatre, where if difficulties arise limb salvage surgery is immediately possible – a concern in the angiography room in the radiology department.

Chapter 7

Diagnostic Angiography

CATHETERS

Catheter size is defined by three methods:

- Length
- Outer diameter – French (Fr) size (calculated by dividing the Fr number by 3, e.g. 6 Fr = 2 mm)
- Inner diameter – this is allied to the guide wire diameter that passes along the catheter

Examples are:

- 5 Fr would be the largest catheter diameter in common use
- 4 Fr provides sufficient stiffness for turning the catheter into selected vessel studies – smaller has less catheter torque strength
- 3 Fr may be used for nonselective vessel work to reduce puncture site size and impact on the patient

Flow rate of catheters is controlled by the catheter size and typically can achieve:

- 3 Fr = 6–8 mL/s
- 4 Fr = 16–18 mL/s
- 5 Fr = 20–25 mL/s

Index of Medical Imaging, First Edition. Jonathan McConnell.
© 2011 Blackwell Publishing Ltd. Published 2011 by Blackwell Publishing Ltd.

Catheters should be flushed regularly to prevent thrombus formation at the tip. In cerebral angiography, blood should flow freely into the flush syringe to avoid introducing air or clots into the cerebral circulation, which would have disastrous consequences. A sharp flushing technique should be used in straight or pigtail catheters with side holes to ensure the end hole is also cleared of thrombus.

Catheter types vary according to the job they do. **Nonselective** side-hole catheters enable large amounts of contrast to be delivered in a bolus. The pigtail type is commonly used and this shape prevents inadvertent catheterisation of small branching vessels that would be damaged with the high-flow contrast meant to be delivered by this type of catheter. Straight side-hole catheters are used in vessels too small to accommodate the pigtail, i.e. under 15 mm across.

Selective catheters may have side holes (not to be used in embolotherapy) but can be used with injection pumps in vessels such as the superior mesenteric artery. End-hole catheters are for hand injection only (use of a pump may cause dissection, plaque dislodgement or simply displace the catheter from its position). Both are shaped to enable clear and easy catheterisation of a vessel. Being individually angled to suit vessel origins from the parent, a review of the diagnostic images will ensure you select the most appropriately angled catheter for the vessel you wish to visualise and/or treat.

Common catheter shapes include:

Nonselective

Pigtail

Straight

Selective

Cobra   Sidewinder   Berenstein

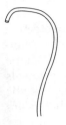 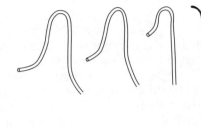 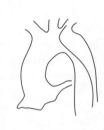

Berenstein catheter with
possible placement
scenario

Renal double   Headhunter
curve (RDC)

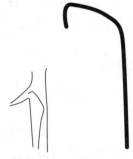 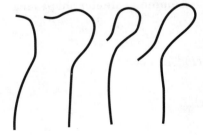

Renal double curve   Headhunter catheters 1, 3, 5 and 6 patterns with
catheter with possible   suggested placement scenarios
placement scenario

GUIDEWIRES

There are several characteristics to consider with guidewires.

Length

Standard length = 140 cm
Longer guidewires = 180 cm or 260 cm

The longer guidewires are used in upper limb work from a groin access, when catheter exchanges are required for visceral, renal or hepatic vessels and when the catheter is over 90 cm or has an angioplasty balloon so that the guide does not disappear down the catheter unexpectedly due to a loss of traction.

Diameter

Range between 0.014 and 0.038 inches
Finer microcatheter work = 0.014–0.018 inches

Tip of wire

The floppy end of the wire tip varies between 1 and 6 cm; shorter ones are better for carotid and hepatic vein work. Tip length is probably best governed by ability to site transition between wire and tip in the target vessel so catheters can be securely passed into these vessels.

Stiffness

Tortuosity and level of disease in an atherosclerotic vessel will dictate 'floppiness' of the wire as this will control an ability to negotiate a way through. Increasing degrees of 'stiffness' are:

- Bentson or movable core wires = **floppy**
- Standard 0.035 J or straight hydrophilic wire = **normal stiffness**
- Stiff hydrophilic, heavy-duty J or straight guidewires = **stiffer**
- Extra stiff wires, Amplatz super anf flexfinder = **stiff**
- Lunderquist (for use in vessel straightening in stent grafting) = **stiffest**

GENERAL ANGIOGRAPHY SET

Arterial puncture needle – 21 gauge for 3 Fr guidewire or 18 gauge for 4 Fr guidewire
For 4 Fr catheter use 150–180 cm 4 Fr guidewire with 3 mm J tip
For 3 Fr catheter use the 3 Fr guidewire usually supplied
Arterial sheath for catheter changes or angioplasty balloon catheter passage

Catheter:

- Pigtail for high flow flush injections
- Straight for small vessel use and if pulled back to the iliac artery, e.g. for pressure measurements

Remember to use the shortest catheter possible to reach the target area:

- 3 Fr flow rates have restricted flow rates e.g. 30 cm straight catheter can deliver 6–8 mL/s
- 4 Fr flow rates are length dependent – 60 cm catheter can deliver up to 18–20 mL/s
- 60 cm 4 Fr = abdominal angiography with femoral approach
- 90 cm 4 Fr = brachial arch aortography or abdominal angiography
- 120 cm 4 Fr = radial approach

Sterile high-pressure connector between catheter and pump for space purposes and maintenance of catheter sterility.

Injector is loaded with 100 mL of 300 mg/mL of nonionic iodine-based contrast. Set maximum pump pressure, delivery amount, contrast medium flow rate and pressure rise time to meet requirements of catheter tolerances and its placement position.

Suggested imaging protocols

Lower limb diagnostic angiography

Projection	Volume of contrast (mL)	Injection rate (mL/s)	Imaging frame rate (fps)	Intensifier field size (cm)	Injection delay (s)	X-ray delay (s)
AP aortoiliac	15	8	2	40		0
Oblique aortoiliac	15	8	2	28		0
AP proximal thigh	10	5	2	40		0
AP distal thigh	10–15	5	1	40		Increase as required
AP calf vessels	10–20	5	1	40		Increase as required
Lateral foot	10–20	5	1	28		Increase as required

Further projections may be used to negotiate prosthetic devices, in the hip and knee and to routinely demonstrate branches of the iliac vessels

Iliac obliques*	15	8	2	40	1.5	0
Profunda oblique**	10–20	5	1	40	0	Increase as required
For focal stenotic lesions#	10–20	5	1	28	0	Increase as required
Lateral foot – Charlie Chaplin##	10–20	5	1	40	0	Increase as required

*Iliac obliques allows full assessment of tortuous vessels – use LAO 25° to show right side and vice versa.
**Profunda oblique the common femoral artery (CFA) hides the origin of the profunda femoris. Raise side of interest 30–50° (RAO 30–50° for right side).
#Focal stenoses try 30° obliques in either direction to bring the lesion into profile so is more clearly revealed.
##Charlie Chaplin to see both feet at same time – place heels together and turn toes out using 40 cm intensifier face.

Arch aortogram

Projection	Volume of contrast (mL)	Injection rate (mL/s)	Imaging frame rate (fps)	Intensifier field size (cm)
LAO 30°	40	18–25	2–4	28–40
LAO 60°	40	18–25	2–4	28–40

Renal angiography

Projection	Volume of contrast (mL)	Injection rate (mL/s)	Imaging frame rate (fps)	Intensifier field size (cm)	Catheter position
AP aortogram	15–20	15	2	40	LV 1
20° oblique	15–20	15	2	28	
Selective	10	5	2	28–20	

In renal transplant situations the following is of value.

Renal transplant angiography

Projection	Volume of contrast (mL)	Injection rate (mL/s)	Imaging frame rate (fps)	Intensifier field size (cm)	Catheter position
AP with obliques	10–15	5	2	28–20	Above renal artery. II centred over renal artery and kidney

Hepatic angiography

Catheter position	Projection	Volume of contrast (mL)	Injection rate (mL/s)	Imaging frame rate (fps)	Intensifier field size (cm)	Length of run (s)
Coeliac axis	AP	32	8	2 → 1	40	To include portal vein = 20
Selective hepatic A	AP + RAO 20°	5–15	Hand	2	20–28	5
Splenic A	AP	20	5	2 → 1	40	To include portal vein = 20

Diagnostic Angiography

Mesenteric angiography

Projection	Volume of contrast (mL)	Injection rate (mL/s)	Imaging frame rate (fps)	Intensifier field size (cm)	Centring
SMA AP	30	6	2 → 1	40	Mid-abdominal
AMA AP	10	Hand	2 → 1	28	Rectosigmoid
IMA RAO 25°	10	Hand	2 → 1	28	Rectosigmoid
IMA LAO 30°	10	Hand	2 → 1	28	Ascending colon + splenic flexure
Coeliac axis	30	Hand	2 → 1	40	Epigastrium
Gastroduodenal A	150	6	2	28	Epigastrium
Left gastric A	8–10	Hand	2	28	Epigastrium

Carotid/cerebral angiography

Projection	Volume of contrast (mL)	Injection rate (mL/s)	Imaging frame rate (fps)	Intensifier field size (cm)	Centring
Arch of aorta LAO 30°	30–40	15–20	2	40–28	Aortic root superiorly
Carotid bifurcation AP + lateral	10	Hand	2	28	Carotid bifurcation anterior to C4
Internal carotid extracranial AP + lateral	10	Hand	2	28–40	Over ipsilateral carotid
Internal carotid intracranial AP + lateral	10	Hand	2→1 for venous	28–40	Lateral skull + Townes view
Vertebral AP + lateral	10	Hand	2→1 for venous	28–40	Intracranial – lateral skull + Townes view

PULMONARY ANGIOGRAPHY

This procedure is rarely performed as multislice spiral CT has superseded the angiographic approach, especially if supported by ventilation/perfusion (V/Q) of nuclear medicine. If immediate diagnosis secondary to cardiopulmonary collapse is required, angiography may be used. Pressures of the pulmonary artery (<50 mm Hg systolic = safe for angiography) or right ventricular end diastolic pressure (RVEDP) >20 mm Hg = unsafe for nonselective pulmonary angiography.

Pulmonary angiography

Projection	Volume of contrast (mL)	Injection rate (mL/s)	Imaging frame rate (fps)	Intensifier field size (cm)
AP	40	20	6	40–28
RAO 30° LAO 30°	10	Hand	2	40–28

Chapter 8

Contrast Media, Emergency Drugs and Reaction Responses

Intravenous contrast media have moved away from the high osmolar (1000–2000 mOsm/kg H$_2$O) ionic varieties to the low osmolar (500–1000 mOsm/kg H$_2$O) nonionic types, resulting in a significant gain in terms of reduced reactions and fatalities without a loss of imaging quality. Severe and very severe reactions are quoted as occurring in 0.2–0.04% and 0.0–0.004% of patients with use of high and low osmolar contrast agents, respectively. Most contrast agents that are administered intravascularly are associated with pain and feelings of warmth plus the potential to generate mild to medium allergic reactions that may include a warm sensation and metallic taste in the mouth, nausea/vomiting, rashes/itching, breathing difficulties to possible respiratory or cardiac arrest.

Patients who may have reacted previously (or have allergies), or those with reduced renal competence due to diabetic drug interactions, or those with liver function abnormalities (as the liver is the alternative excretory pathway to the kidneys) may be more susceptible to reactions that could develop to full anaphylactic shock and collapse, or may be susceptible to renal lactic acidosis to generate acute renal failure.

In all patients, prior hydration is a good technique to adopt to protect the kidney. Some departments may favour prophylactic administration of the drug acetylcysteine which is believed to work as a vasodilating oxygen radical scavenger. Diabetic patients

Index of Medical Imaging, First Edition. Jonathan McConnell.
© 2011 Blackwell Publishing Ltd. Published 2011 by Blackwell Publishing Ltd.

being treated with metformin should suspend taking the drug, if not before then for the 48 hours after receipt of contrast media, to reduce the risk of overloading the kidney and inducing renal lactic acidosis. In all cases post-injection hydration is good policy. With patients above 60 years of age, establishing serum creatinine

Iodinated intravascular contrast media

Contrast medium	Brand name	Areas of use
Iohexol (low osmolar nonionic)	Omnipaque 140, 210, 240, 300, 350	Vascular studies Body scanning enhancement Excretion urography (all groups) Arthrography studies Oral gastrointestinal studies
Iopamidol (low osmolar nonionic)	Isovue 128, 200, 300, 370	Vascular studies CT enhancement Excretion urography (all groups) Urography
Iopamidol (low osmolar nonionic)	Niopam 200, 300, 370	Vascular studies Body and brain CT scanning enhancement Myelography Cholangiopancreatography Excretion urography (all groups) Oral gastrointestinal studies Arthrography studies
Iopromide (low osmolar nonionic)	Ultravist 150, 240, 300, 370	Vascular studies Coronary arteriography Body and brain CT scanning enhancement Excretion urography
Ioversol (low osmolar nonionic)	Optiray 160, 240, 300, 320, 350	Vascular studies Body scanning enhancement Excretion urography (all groups)

levels or glomerular filtration rate (GFr) helps identify possible renal impairment and enables the practitioner to ascertain whether the intravascular approach should be taken. Diabetic patients with a serum creatinine level of 4.5 mg/dL or above are highly likely to experience acute renal failure (ARF).

Osmolarity value	Notable side effects or contraindications
322–844 mOsm/kg H₂O (1.1–3 × normal blood value)	Omnipaque 140 and 350 mg I/mL NOT FOR intrathecal use Long-term contact of blood with contrast medium may generate embolisms – could cause stroke or MI – not commonly fatal Transient diarrhoea or nausea with large oral volumes No breast feeding for 24 h post-injection
Isovue 200 onwards range 413–796 mOsm/ kg H₂O	Isovue 200 onwards NOT FOR intrathecal use Not known if excreted in breast milk – suggest no breast feeding for 24 h post-injection May promote renal lactic acidosis in compromised patients
413, 616 and 796 mOsm/kg H₂O	Problems noted with interactions of antipsychotic drugs, antidepressants, glucocorticoids and hypotension-producing agents Transient diarrhoea or nausea with large oral volumes No breast feeding for 24 h post-injection
328, 483, 607, 774 mOsm/kg H₂O	NOT FOR intrathecal use DO NOT mix Ultravist with other drugs Not known if excreted in breast milk – suggest no breast feeding for 24 h post-injection Cease biguanides (metformin) 48 h each side of examination if possible
Optiray 160 onwards range 355–792 mOsm/ kg H₂O	NOT FOR intrathecal use Not known if excreted in breast milk – suggest no breast feeding for 24 h post-injection

(Continued)

Media, Drugs and Reaction Responses

Contrast medium	Brand name	Areas of use
Ioxaglate Meglumine, Ioxaglate Sodium (low osmolar ionic)	Hexabrix	Vascular studies Coronary arteriography Body and brain CT scanning enhancement Excretion urography Hysterosalpingography Arthrography
Metrizamide	Amipaque 170, 300	Vascular studies Brain CT enhancement Retrograde cystourethrography and pyelography Splenoportography Hysterosalpingography Cholangiography Myelography

Oral or gastrointestinal lumen contrast media

Contrast medium	Brand name	Areas of use
Sodium, meglumine amidotrizoate	Gastrografin	Gastrointestinal tract investigations orally or as an enema
Barium sulphate (oral or rectal)	Entero-Vu	Digestive system radiography
Barium sulphate (dry oral preparation, add water)	E-Z Cat Dry (oral)	Digestive system radiography
Barium Sulphate (premixed solution oral or rectal application)	Readi-Cat Polibar + (plus) Polibar rapid	Digestive system radiography or diluted as contrast media for CT abdominal scanning

Osmolarity value	Notable side effects or contraindications
600 mOsm/kg H$_2$O	NOT FOR intrathecal use Not known if excreted in breast milk – suggest no breast feeding for 24 h post-injection When used with GA, increased reactions noted due to extended circulation times and contact with contrast agent Strong allergic history may require prophylactic antihistamine or corticosteroid use Avoid dehydration
Osmolarity values across these contrast media range 300–484 mOsm/kg H$_2$O	Problems noted with interactions of antipsychotic drugs, antidepressants, glucocorticoids and hypotension-producing agents Known passage of metrizamide into breast milk at 1 mg over 2 days

Osmolarity value	Notable side effects or contraindications
215 mOsm/ kg H$_2$O	DO NOT USE in cases of hyperparathyroid disease NOT FOR intravascular use Dehydrated and patients with known allergy to iodine should not be exposed to gastrografin: H$_2$O and electrolytes should be balanced before use Not known if excreted in breast milk – suggest no breast feeding for 24 h post-exposure
	DO NOT use in gastrointestinal perforation or infectious gastroenteritis Contraindicated in dehydration, diverticulitis of gastrointestinal tract, dysphagia, gastrointestinal obstruction, predisposition to aspiration, ulcerative colitis Adverse effects: Commonest: abdominal pain with cramps, constipation, diarrhoea Rarely: abdominal swelling, acute abdominal pain, allergic reactions, anaphylaxis, dyspnoea, faecal impaction, nausea, vomiting NO KNOWN RISKS with lactation as is not absorbed
	As per Entero-Vu
	As per Entero-Vu

Media, Drugs and Reaction Responses

Other drugs used in the radiology department

Drug	Brand name	Areas of use	Concentration	Notable side effects/comments
Hyoscine-N-butylbromide (injection as an antispasmodic)	Buscopan	Involuntary muscle antispasmodic/anticholinergic – used mainly in barium enema, CT colonography, abdominal MRI to enhance image quality	1 ampoule intramuscular = 20 mg	May cause dry throat and mouth, dizziness, eye blurring (NOTE: DO NOT USE in patients with glaucoma, megacolon, porphyria or myasthenic gravis), arrhythmia, flushing or fainting. Related to scopolamine (truth serum) and atropine. May cause constipation +/– paralytic ileus if used with opioids or antiperistaltic drugs
Metoclopramide (additive to oral contrast medium)	Maxolon	Intestinal prokinetic (also has antiemetic uses)		Used to aid peristalsis in duodenum and jejunum so aid gastric emptying and is often an additive for Barium meal + followthrough. Not for use in cases of phaeochromocytoma (adrenal gland tumour) or Parkinson's disease (as may worsen condition). Longer-term therapy causes more severe effects including oculogyric crisis (rolling of the eyes), hyper- and hypotension or supraventricular tachycardia

Sedation and analgesia in radiology

The use of sedation and analgesia in radiological examinations is widespread. The aims of its use include control of unwanted motor behaviour so examination performance is not interfered with, to reduce sympathetic nervous system responses such as hypertension/tachycardia and reduce anxiety, cause amnesia, sedate the patient and provide analgesia. These should be achieved with quick and predictable recovery.

The use of these drugs requires full consent to be obtained, which is likely to begin through the referral process for procedures with the patient, parents/guardians or family/carers. Departments should be equipped with similar arrangements to operating theatres with tipping trolleys, crash carts and call systems that are accessible and familiar to all staff involved with their potential use. Out-of-hours procedures are the most risky as patients may be critically ill, have other morbidities and there may be a lack of appropriate nursing or anaesthetic support. Without these being in place it is ill advised to go ahead with procedures of this nature. Monitoring equipment should be able to automatically measure heart rate and blood pressure and provide pulse oximetry with continuous electrocardiography. Sedation level should be continuously monitored every 5 minutes once a stable sedation level is achieved.

Analgesics are administered prior to sedation, should pain be expected after the procedure. Paracetamol (oral or intravenous) is given 30–60 minutes before, supplemented with nonsteroidal anti-inflammatory drugs (NSAIDs) relative to renal capability of patients. Oxygen support at 2–4 L/min via nasal prongs or face mask is advised for any procedures other than light sedation, and preoxygenation should be provided if opioids or benzodiazepines are expected to be used. Sedatives should be delivered in small increments with sufficient time between doses to allow the drugs to act before giving the next dose. Irritability and agitation could represent poor brain oxygenation or airway obstruction rather than insufficient sedation: **keep checking the patient**. Drug doses should be calculated according to age, body size, drug absorption and administration mode, comorbidities, interactions with regular medications or other sedatives/narcotics.

Sedatives, analgesics and anaesthetics in radiology (arranged
according to preferences)

Name	Concentration	Onset time + duration
Common local anaesthetics		
Lidocaine/ lignocaine	0.5–5% 1% most common use	2–5 mins 1 hour action 3 hours if + adrenaline mix
Bupivicaine	0.25–0.75% +/– adrenaline 0.25% most common use	5–10 mins 3 hour action (if + adrenaline duration will increase)
Common simple analgesias		
Paracetamol	500 mg per tablet	30–60 mins 4–6 hours action
Ibuprofen (NSAID)	200–600 mg tablets	30–60 mins 4–6 hours action
Common opioids used in analgesia and sedation		
Fentanyl	25 µg increments	2–3 mins 30–60 min action
Morphine	2–5 mg increments	5–20 mins 4–8 hours action
Pethidine		5–20 mins Shorter action time than morphine, half-life 120–150 mins
Benzodiazepines used in sedation		
Midazolam	5 mg/mL injection 7.5 and 15 mg tablets	1–3 mins 1 hour action

Maximum dose	Notable side effects/comments
3 mg/kg (300 mg) 7 mg/kg (500 mg) if + adrenaline	High doses = central nervous system toxicity to produce periorbital tingling, seizure and coma
2 mg/kg (150 mg) 3 mg/kg (225 mg) if + adrenaline	Highly cardiotoxic – causes arrhythmias. AVOID IV delivery Good for use when post-procedure pain expected
4 g daily 500–1000 mg every 4–6 h	
0.8–2.4 g daily 200–600 mg every 4–6 h	Avoid use in asthmatics or gastric problems, e.g. peptic bleeding, reflux. Nausea is a noted side effect; ensure no contraindications with other drugs being used
1–2 µg/kg induces analgesia	Usually IV delivery but oral and transdermal possible Causes dizziness and apnoea in high doses Respiratory depression is up to 4 h after analgesia has worn off. Observe ventilation and oxygenation throughout Naxolone (Narcan) should be available to reverse effects
IM or subcutaneous delivery	Nausea, vomiting and dizziness Sedation and respiratory depression are extended in renally impaired due to accumulation of morphine in the kidney
25–100 mg IV or IM Administer every 4–6 h	Nausea, vomiting and dizziness as well as respiratory depression and hypotension are sequelae to excessive dosage
Give in 0.5–1 mg increments until titrated effect reached 0.5 mg/kg as oral premedication Paediatric effective doses Intranasal 0.2 mg/kg also use with analgesic for painful exams Oral 0.5 mg/kg in under 8 years, poor results in older children Rectal 0.3–0.6 mg/kg	Use with atorvastatin causes reduced elimination rate of midazolam – check other drugs for interactions that may speed up or inhibit metabolism Favoured paediatric sedative as there is a wide range of delivery options Elderly, COPD patients and combination with CNS depressants e.g. alcohol and tricyclic antidepressants expose individuals to greater reactions. Flumazenil is the antagonist to midazolam and will reverse overdose effects. Nystagmus, hypotension, ataxia, somnolence and respiratory arrest are typical symptoms of overdose

Media, Drugs and Reaction Responses

(Continued)

Name	Concentration	Onset time + duration
Diazepam	5 mg tablets 5 mg/mL for IV/IM injection	2–3 mins Up to 6 hours
Reversal drugs		
Flumazenil	500 µg/5 mL	Duration 15–140 mins
Naloxone (Narcan)	0.4–2 mg Narcan though 0.1–0.2 mg titrated according to required reversal effect for respiratory depression	1 min action 45 mins duration

Emergency drugs

Name	Action	Indications
Key drugs that may be found on the emergency trolley		
Adenosine	Decreases conduction through the AV node	Conversion to sinus rhythm from paroxysmal supraventricular tachycardia
Amiodarone	Anti – arrhythmia drug to inhibit potassium outflow channels of the conducting tissue of the heart and prolong polarisation.	Treatment of refractory ventricular fibrillation, pulseless ventricular tachycardia (VT), haemodynamically stable VT and other resistant tachycardia
Aminophylline	Eases breathing by relaxing airway's smooth muscle	Relieves symptoms of bronchospasm/asthma

Media, Drugs and Reaction Responses

Maximum dose	Notable side effects/comments
1–2 mg increments titrated to effect per patient is advised	DO NOT USE in patients acutely intoxicated with narcotics or alcohol, those with renal or hepatic disorders, pregnant or breast feeding women and those with known benzodiazepine allergies. Flumazenil is the antidote to diazepam
0.2 mg every 60–120 seconds until effect seen. Continue to maximum of 3 mg per hour	Where the duration time is being exceeded, airway support may be required as an adjunct to close observation and continuous infusion of flumazenil
0.4–2 mg until effect evident – 10 mg indicates effects not due to narcotic poisoning. Child's dose = 0.01 mg/kg	Hypo- and hypertension, ventricular tachycardia, ventricular fibrillation, dyspnoea, pulmonary oedema, cardiac arrest Abrupt opioid reversal may result in nausea, vomiting, sweating and tachycardia with extension as indicated above

Side effects	Contraindications/notes
Facial flushing, dyspnoea, hyperventilation and dizziness are reported side effects	6 mg rapid IV dose ideally via CVP line. Give 12 mg follow-up dose if SVT not rectified. A further 12 mg dose may be used
Hypotension Sinus arrest Bronchospasm	Best administered by central venous catheter if present. An initial bolus dose of 300 mg over 5–15 minutes into a peripheral vein is suggested for cardiac arrest with 300 mg infused over the next hour
Arrhythmias, respiratory arrest	Active peptic ulcer disease (not a major concern during respiratory distress!)

(Continued)

Name	Action	Indications
Atropine	Blocks action of vagus nerve on sinoatrial and atrioventricular node to increase conduction velocity. The AV refractory period is decreased thus increasing heart rate	Use following adrenaline in asystole or low heart rates under 60 bpm
Bumetanide	Promotes excretion of sodium and water	Pulmonary oedema in heart failure, hepatic or renal disease
Calcium Gluconate	Replaces and maintains Ca^{2+} to raise serum Ca^{2+}	Treats hypocalcaemic emergency/tetany/supports cardiac arrest and magnesium intoxification
Diazepam	Anticonvulsant, reduces anxiety and spasm/seizures to promote calmness/ sleep	Anxiety and therefore cardiac stress or as preprocedural sedation. Adjunct in seizure/status epilepticus
Diclofenac Sodium	Relieves inflammation, pain and fever	Potent analgesic NSAID for musculoskeletal pain post-trauma
Diphenhydramine Hydrochloride	Relieves allergy symptoms to promote calmness and sleep	Allergy symptoms and suppresses coughs, generates a calming effect
Epinephrine (Adrenaline) 1 : 1000	Bronchial smooth muscle relaxant; cardiac muscle stimulant; decreases pain; stops local bleeding	Bronchospasm, anaphylaxis, haemostasis, restoration of cardiac rhythm post-arrest

Side effects	Contraindications/notes
Single large dose may cause palpitations, dilated pupils, hot dry skin, thirst, dizziness, tremor, restlessness, fatigue and ataxia	No absolute proof that has any value in asystole; anecdotal accounts in grave situations suggests unlikely to be harmful in asystole events
Renal failure, thrombocytopenia in extended therapy	Anuria/hepatic coma, severe electrolyte depletion are other side effects More potent alternative to fruse-mide (diuretic)
Bradycardia, arrhythmias and cardiac arrest	Ventricular fibrillation, hypercalcaemia, hypophosphataemia, renal calculi, sarcoidosis, renal failure, cardiac disease, patients on digitalis (digoxin)
Bradycardia +/– cardiovascular collapse, respiratory depression. If overused, withdrawal symptoms	Child under 6/12, shock, coma, alcohol intoxication, early pregnancy or breast feeding, hepatic or renally impaired, elderly or debilitated patients
Heart failure, acute renal failure, laryngeal oedema	Asthma, urticaria, hepatic porphyria
Seizures, thrombocytopenia, shock	Acute asthma
Cerebral haemorrhage/cerebral vascular accident (raised BP), ventricular fibrillation/shock	Shock, organic brain damage, arrhythmia, cardiac insufficiency

Media, Drugs and Reaction Responses

(Continued)

Name	Action	Indications
Esmolol Hydrochloride	Antiarrhythmic – restores normal cardiac rhythm	Supraventricular tachycardia; controls ventricular rate in atrial fibrillation
Heparin Sodium	Anticoagulant	Deep vein thrombosis/ pulmonary embolism. Maintains indwelling catheter patency
Hydrocortisone	Reduces inflammation	Treats severe inflammation, shock and adrenal insufficiency
Lignocaine	Sodium channel blocker with antiarrhythmic effects	Ventricular fibrillation of pulseless ventricular tachycardia
Magnesium sulphate	Necessary for membrane stability	Myocardial hyperexcitability with raised potassium/digoxin levels. Use with ventricular fibrillation of pulseless ventricular tachycardia
Naloxone (Narcan)		Opioid overdose
Potassium chloride	Necessary for membrane stability	Low potassium + low magnesium + digoxin may cause life-threatening cardiac arrhythmias
Sodium bicarbonate	Combats acidosis through a buffering mechanism	Evidence of cardiac arrhythmias. Arterial blood gases or pH > 7.1 increases cardiac risk

Side effects	Contraindications/notes
Hypotension and bronchospasm, tissue necrosis in extravasation	Sinus bradycardia, >1st degree heart block, cardiogenic shock or overwhelming heart failure, kidney function ↓, diabetes, bronchospasm
Haemorrhage, thrombocytopenia (low platelet count) due to heparin action	Active bleeding, ? intracerebral haemorrhage, excessively denuded skin, open ulcerative wounds
Heart failure, arrhythmias and thromboembolism	Recent myocardial infarction, diastolic murmur, osteoporosis
Slurred speech, altered consciousness, seizures and muscle twitching. Hypotension, heart block and bradycardia possible	Limited studies available to guide practice
Flushing, sweating, sharply lowered blood pressure, hypothermia, stupor and respiratory depression	Little data exists for or against its use during cardiac arrest
Hypo- and hypertension, ventricular tachycardia, ventricular fibrillation, dyspnoea, pulmonary oedema, cardiac arrest	Abrupt opioid reversal may result in nausea, vomiting, sweating and tachycardia with extension as indicated opposite
Use may generate hyperkalaemia (high serum potassium) + hypotension and/or asystole. Tissue necrosis from extravasation	
Overdose results in hyper-irritability and tetanus though this is noted for longer-term treatments rather than emergency situations	Only recommended where arrest has continued for 10–15 minutes and arterial blood gases suggest metabolic acidosis is present

Media, Drugs and Reaction Responses

Routines for reactions to radiographic contrast media

<table>
<tr><td></td><td>**Reaction description**</td><td>**Level**</td><td>**Notes**</td></tr>
<tr><td colspan="4">*Low level reactions*</td></tr>
<tr><td rowspan="2">MINOR REACTION NOT LIFE-THREATENING</td><td>Nausea/ vomiting</td><td>Transient:
Protracted:</td><td>Supportive treatment
Consider use of an antiemetic, provide support</td></tr>
<tr><td>Urticaria</td><td>Scattered and transient
Protracted and scattered

Profound</td><td>Observe with supportive treatment
Use of appropriate antihistamine IM or IV. Observe for drowsiness +/− hypotension
Consider adrenaline 1 : 1000 0.1–0.3 mL (0.1–0.3 mg) IM in adults. Paediatrics use 0.01 mg/kg IM up to 0.3 mg maximum. Repeat as needed</td></tr>
<tr><td colspan="4">*High level reactions*</td></tr>
<tr><td rowspan="3">MEDIUM TO SEVERE REACTION MAY BE LIFE-THREATENING IF NOT TREATED PROMPTLY</td><td>Bronchospasm</td><td colspan="2">1. Oxygen by mask 6–10 L/min
2. β2 agonist (terbutaline, albuterol, metaproteranol) metered dose 2–3 deep inhalations
3. Adrenaline:
Normal BP = 1 : 1000 0.1–0.3 mL (0.1–0.3 mg) for adults (reduce dose if coronary artery disease or elderly)
Paediatrics use 0.01 mg/kg to 0.3 mg maximum
Low BP = 1 : 1000 0.5 mL (0.5 mg) for adults: Paediatrics 0.01 mg/kg IM)</td></tr>
<tr><td>Laryngeal oedema</td><td colspan="2">1. Oxygen by mask 6–10 L/min
2. IM adrenaline 1 : 1000, 0.5 mL (0.5 mg) repeated as necessary</td></tr>
<tr><td>Hypotension</td><td colspan="2">**Isolated hypotension**
1. Elevate patient's legs
2. Oxygen by mask 6–10 L/min
3. Rapid IV fluid – normal saline or lactated Ringer's solution
Vagal reaction (bradycardia + hypotension)
1. Elevate patient's legs
2. Oxygen by mask 6–10 L/min
3. Atropine 0.6–1.0 mg IV, repeat if necessary after 3–5 mins to 3 mg total (0.04 mg/kg) in adults
Paediatrics = 0.02 mg/kg IV (maximum 0.6 mg per dose), repeat if necessary to 2 mg total
4. Rapid IV fluid – normal saline or lactated Ringer's solution</td></tr>
</table>

Media, Drugs and Reaction Responses

	Reaction description	Level	Notes
SEVERE REACTION LIFE-THREATENING	*Generalised anaphylactoid reaction*		
	1. Call resuscitation team 2. Suction airway as required and begin basic life support 3. If hypotensive elevate legs 4. Oxygen by mask 6–10 l/min 5. IM adrenaline (1:1000), 0.5 mL (0.5 mg) in adults. Repeat as needed. In paediatrics 0.01 mg/kg to 0.3 mg maximum dose 6. IV fluids – normal saline or lactated Ringer's solution 7. H1-antihistamine e.g. diphenhydramine 25–50 mg IV 8. β2-agonist metered dose inhaler for persistent bronchospasm: 2 or 3 deep inhalations		

References

Hand H. and Banks A. (2004) The contents of the resuscitation trolley. *Nursing Standard* 18(44): 43–52.

Jensen S.C. and Peppers M.P. (2006) *Pharmacology and Drug Administration for Imaging Technologists* 2nd Ed. Mosby/Elsevier, St Louis, MO.

Patatas K. and Koukkoulli A. (2009) The use of sedation in the radiology department. *Clinical Radiology* 64: 655–663.

Starkey E. and Sammons H.M. (2010) Sedation for radiological imaging. *Archives of Disease in Childhood Education and Practice.* doi:10.1136/adc.2008.153072. Published online and accessed 3 August 2010.

Thomsen H.S. and Morcos S.K. (2004) Management of acute adverse reactions to contrast media. *European Radiology* 14(3): 476–481.

Media, Drugs and Reaction Responses

Chapter 9

Computed Tomography Protocols

Assume adult unless otherwise stated.

COMPUTED TOMOGRAPHY OF BRAIN AND HEAD

Performed to exclude a specific pathology or trauma, CT examinations of the brain and regions of the head are generally used to investigate causes for presentation of multiple clinical manifestations. Intravenous contrast media may be employed, though not in all cases. However, when lesions are best revealed with contrast agent, scans are performed initially without contrast, then repeated after contrast administration.

Index of Medical Imaging, First Edition. Jonathan McConnell.
© 2011 Blackwell Publishing Ltd. Published 2011 by Blackwell Publishing Ltd.

Brain: pathologies and indications

Tumours	Vascular	Infectious	Degenerative
• astrocytoma • craniopharyngioma • glioblastoma • glioma • haemangioblastoma • medulloblastoma • meningioma • metastases • neurinoma • oligodendroglioma • plexus papilloma	• arteriovenous malformation (AVM) • aneurysm • infarction • ischaemia	• abscess • encephalitis • meningitis • tuberculosis	• cerebral atrophy • hydrocephalus • multiple sclerosis

Trauma	Bleeding	Other	Indications
• cerebral contusion • fracture • pneumatocele	• extradural • subarachnoid • subdural (acute/chronic) • parenchymal • petechial	• subarachnoid cysts • subdural hygroma	• cerebrovascular attack • dementia screen • headache • MRI contraindicated/not available • transient ischaemic attack

Brain: window width (WW) and window level (WL) viewing values

Window	Width (HU)	Level (HU)
Bone range all skull	2000–3000	200–500
Soft tissue post fossa	100–160	30–40
Soft tissue cerebral vault	70–90	30–40
Blood	80	80

Head: sequence protocol for multislice scanners

Acquisition	No of detectors and width	Reconstruction thickness/ interval (mm)	mAs	kV	Algorithm	Rotation time	IV contrast
Axial sequence	16 × 0.6 mm	5 mm/5 mm	~250	140	soft tissue	1.0 second	if indicated

Scan from base of skull to vertex with angulation from skull base to superior orbital margin. For those patients who cannot be scanned without irradiation of the orbital region, the gantry may be tilted and scanning in sequence mode adopted. The sequence technique often reduces radiation dose compared with helical volume approaches. On newer scanners, sequence scanning is as fast as helical. Multiplanar reconstructions (MPRs) can also be created from sequence data acquisition but, because the slice data is not overlapping, some stair-step artefact is present. This can only be avoided by using a helical technique with thinner detector sizes, so creating a true volumetric data set.

Head: multislice spiral/helical protocol

Acquisition	No of detectors and width	Reconstruction thickness/ interval (mm)	mAs	kV	Algorithm	Rotation time	IV contrast
Axial helical	64 × 0.5 mm	1 mm/0.5 mm	~200	140	soft tissue	1.0 second	if indicated

Adult head: MPR planes, thickness and intervals

MPRs	Slice thickness	Slice interval
Axial	5 mm	5 mm
Coronal	5 mm	5 mm
Sagittal	5 mm	5 mm

Computed Tomography Protocols

Following IV contrast administration, volume data acquisition permits brain vessel delineation in multiple planes of a standard approaching subtraction angiography without the invasive approach. If used as a cerebral angiogram replacement technique, the arterial phase can be obtained with an 8 or 12 second delay or contrast bolus tracking software. If thinner slices are required these can be recreated using MPRs without having to rescan the patient. Helical (volume) data sets produce higher quality MPRs as long as thin overlapping slices are used when compared with sequence approaches.

Computed tomography of orbits

Data is usually obtained in the axial plane only following intravenous contrast in orbital examinations (non-contrast scans may be done but remember the radiation dose to the lens) with MPRs created in coronal and sagittal planes. To see the optic nerve and canal, oblique axial MPRs can be created according to need from the clinical indication.

Orbit: pathologies and indications

Benign tumours	• cavernous angiomas • optic nerve gliomas • optic nerve sheath meningiomas • sphenoid meningiomas	Malignant tumours	• lacrimal gland tumours • lymphomas • metastases • primary carcinomas	Inflammatory lesions	• mucocoeles • myositis • pseudotumours • pyocoeles
Traumatic lesions	• carotid-cavernous fistula • fracture • retrobulbar haematomas	Other	• abscess • foreign bodies	Indications	• exophthalmos • MRI contraindicated or not available • proptosis • suspected mass • visual disturbances

Orbits: multislice spiral/helical protocol

Acquisition	No of detectors and width	Reconstruction thickness/ interval (mm)	mAs	kV	Algorithm	Rotation time	IV contrast
Axial helical	16 × 0.75 mm	1 mm/0.5 mm	~150	120	soft tissue	0.5–1.0 second	✓

Orbits: MPR planes, thickness and intervals

MPRs soft tissue	Slice thickness	Slice interval
Axial	3 mm	3 mm
Coronal	3 mm	3 mm
Sagittal	3 mm	3 mm

Computed tomography of facial bones

Facial CT requires an acquisition from the upper teeth (maxillary margin) to 1 cm above the frontal sinus which is defined on the scout view. MPRs can be generated in other planes from this data set.

Facial bones: multislice spiral/helical protocol

Acquisition	No of detectors and width	Reconstruction thickness/ interval (mm)	mAs	kV	Algorithm	Rotation time	IV contrast
Axial helical	64 × 0.5 mm	1 mm/0.5 mm	~150	120	soft tissue and bone	0.5 second	X

Facial bones: MPR planes, thickness and intervals, bone reconstructions

MPRs bone	Slice thickness	Slice interval
Axial	1 mm	2 mm
Coronal	1 mm	2 mm
Sagittal	1 mm	2 mm

Computed Tomography Protocols

Facial bones: MPR planes, thickness and intervals, soft tissue reconstructions (if required)

MPRs soft tissue	Slice thickness	Slice interval
Axial	3 mm	3 mm
Coronal	3 mm	3 mm
Sagittal	3 mm	3 mm

To improve fine bone detail and enhance the signal-to-noise ratio in the thin slices necessary for facial bone fracture evaluation an increased exposure may be necessary. Soft-tissue viewing algorithms are used with MPRs to create 3D volume-rendered (3D VR) images. In combination these approaches will reveal fat surrounding the inferior rectus muscles that herniates through the orbital floor in fractures. 3D VR allows a relational understanding of facial fractures not feasible on plain radiographs.

Computed tomography of paranasal sinuses

Paranasal sinus: pathologies and indications

Tumours	• osteomas • viscerocranial carcinomas	Congenital	• hypoplasia and aplasia	Inflammation	• mucocoeles • pyocoele • sinusitis
Other	• fracture • fungal infections • nasal polyposis	Indications	• complex infection • suspected mass		

Paranasal sinuses: WW and WL viewing values

Window	Width (HU)	Level (HU)
Bone	1500–3000	200–500
Soft tissue range	200–400	30–100

Paranasal sinuses: multislice spiral/helical protocol

Acquisition	No of detectors and width	Reconstruction thickness/ interval (mm)	mAs	kV	Algorithm	Rotation time	IV contrast
Range 1: axial helical	32 × 0.625 mm	0.625 mm/0.5 mm	150–200	120	bone	0.5–1.0 second	X

Facial bones: MPR planes, thickness and intervals

MPRs	Slice thickness	Slice interval
Axial	0.5–1 mm	1–2 mm
Coronal	0.5–1 mm	1–2 mm
Sagittal	0.5–1 mm	1–2 mm

Computed tomography of temporal bone

Temporal bone: pathologies and indications

Tumours	• acoustic neurinomas • glomus tumours • primary and secondary malignant tumours	Congenital	• dysplasias of the middle ear, inner ear and ossicles • stenosis and atresia of the external auditory canal	Inflammation	• malignant external otitis • otitis media and mastoiditis
Other	• anomalies of blood vessels and nerves • cholesteatoma • fracture	Indications	• hearing deficits • MRI contraindicated/ not available • vertigo		

Temporal bone:WW and WL viewing values

Window	Width (HU)	Level (HU)
Bone	3000–4000	500–1000
Soft tissue	100–160	30–40

Include from the inferior mastoid edge to the most superior margin of mastoid air cells. Reconstructions in other planes are taken from the volumetric data set. Often only bone reconstructions are imaged on bone windows for review; soft tissue reconstructions and windows are mentioned here as they may be clinically indicated.

Internal auditory meatus: multislice spiral/helical protocol

Acquisition	No of detectors and width	Reconstruction thickness/ interval (mm)	mAs	kV	Algorithm	Rotation time	IV contrast
Axial helical	32 × 0.625 mm	0.625 mm/0.625 mm	~200	120	bone	0.5–1.0 second	if indicated

Internal auditory meatus: MPR planes, thickness and intervals

MPRs	Slice thickness	Slice interval
Axial	0.625 mm	0.625 mm
Coronal	0.625 mm	0.625 mm
Sagittal	0.625 mm when done	0.625 mm when done

Direct coronal scanning is no longer required as small-slice collimation enables coronal MPRs to be created from the volumetric data set. By reducing the pitch (table feed per rotation), data collection is increased, thus minimising stair-stepping artefacts in MPRs.

Computed tomography of the pituitary fossa

MRI is the modality of choice for pituitary investigations. Pre and post IV contrast scan performance is normal about 20 seconds post injection using 50 mL of contrast at 2 mL/sec. Presenting with other endocrine complaints, pituitary scans are performed to demonstrate micro and macro tumours (adenomas) with thin-slice MPRs generated from the volume data set. Axial coronal and sagittal planes are the usual reconstruction requirements.

Computed tomography of the paediatric brain

Similar considerations apply in terms of sequence or helical/ volume acquisition as noted in the adult discussion, though note well that paediatric doses are greater from the lower radiation filtering effect due to smaller body size. MRI may be a more appropriate examination but CT has value post trauma, after operation and in evaluation of hydrocephalus and ventricular-peritoneal shunt function/integrity. The same basic method of scanning is employed but with exposure ranges and IV contrast media volumes designed to account for patients of specific age, weight and size, to minimise radiation and contrast load to the immature physiology.

Paediatric head: sequence multislice protocol

Acquisition	No of detectors and width	Reconstruction thickness/ interval (mm)	mAs	kV	Algorithm	Rotation time	IV contrast
Axial sequence	16 × 1.2 mm	5 mm/5 mm	~200 or lower	140	soft tissue	1.0 second	if indicated

Paediatric brain: WW and WL viewing values (HU)

Age	0–5 years		6–13 years		14–17 years	
Window	Width	Level	Width	Level	Width	Level
Bone all skull	2000	500	2000	500	2000	500
Soft tissue post fossa	90–160	30–40	90–130	35	100–150	35
Soft tissue cerebral vault	70–90	30–40	70	35	70	35

COMPUTED TOMOGRAPHY OF SPINE AND NECK

Identification of the correct vertebral level is essential when scanning differing spinal areas. DO NOT label specific vertebrae, as your mis-identification can cause the wrong level to be operated on; this is especially true if the report is not linked to the images, which the radiologist may have identified differently. An error such as this will be retained on the images. Alternatively provide scout images with and without scan prescription lines so the viewer makes the correct association; many machines make it possible to include an appropriately identified scout with a single line imprinted upon it to match with the linked axial image.

AP and lateral scout images can both be employed so that the exact level to which the axial image relates is clear to the viewer. Be certain you are scanning the requested vertebrae when establishing traumatic changes; a scout of the entire spinal region will help with this. If scanning a soft-tissue neck examination ask the patient not to swallow, and to breathe quietly. Swallowing will generate blurring to imitate pathology such as an abscess. Beware of metal in head holders if you use one for neck examinations, as this will generate artefacts, rendering the scan useless.

Positioning for spine/neck examinations

Topogram	Examination	Patient positioning
Axial lateral topogram/ scout (to include entire neck)	axial cervical spine axial neck	• use head holder • patient positioned supine, head first • arms by patient's side or across chest • use Velcro straps and immobilisation pads to help the patient keep his/her head still • if the patient is likely to jump off table use thick Velcro straps and strap the patient down to the table for safety • get patient to relax shoulders to decrease artefact • ensure that patient is comfortable
Axial AP and lateral topogram/scout (to include vertebrae under investigation)	axial lumbar spine axial thoracic spine	• use black carbon fibre head holder or table extension (for feet) with pillow placed on it, patient positioned supine, feet first • arms raised above patient's head • if patient liable to jump off table use thick Velcro strap and strap the patient to the table for safety • ensure that patient is comfortable by placing a large wedge sponge under their knees

Computed tomography of neck

The following table outlines typical pathologies and clinical presentations that require CT of the neck.

Neck: pathologies and indications

Pathologies	• abscess • carcinoma • fracture • goitre	Indications	• difficulty in swallowing • hoarse voice • lymphadenopathy • retrosternal thyroid extension • trauma

Neck CT imaging extends from the base of the skull/hard palate until the aortic arch. Where pathology focuses on the thyroid gland, check the need for iodinated contrast agents. Uptake of iodine from this source prevents iodine-based radiotherapy for as much as 8 weeks as the thyroid cannot receive more iodine. When iodine-based contrast can be used the flow rate and volume is in the order of 75–100 mL at 2 mL per second. With thyroid goitres, consider an extended scan range into the mediastinum to fully evaluate retrosternal presentations. Where the vocal cord is involved, thin MPRs may be necessary to delineate tumours from other anatomy that may be invaded. Amalgam fillings can produce artefacts, which can obscure some of the anatomy within the neck.

Contrast monitoring software, using opacification of the carotid artery as the trigger to show strong artery and vein uptake, is helpful when evaluating the neck. A 30 mL hand-injected bolus is given in some centres to aid highlighting of the neck musculature. Alternatively a 2 mL/sec flow rate is delivered by pump with later triggering of the scan to show the neck arteries and veins. A dual-phase injection is an alternative approach where the first bolus is delivered during scout image generation and a later injection given with a 25–30 sec delay before beginning to scan.

Neck: WW and WL viewing values

Window	Width (HU)	Level (HU)
Soft tissue	250–500	30–60

Neck: multislice spiral/helical protocol

Acquisition	No of detectors and width	Reconstruction thickness/ interval (mm)	mAs	kV	Algorithm	Rotation time	IV contrast
Axial helical	64 × 0.625 mm	0.625/0.625 mm	~200 modulated	120	soft tissue	0.5–1.0 second	✓

Neck: MPR planes, thickness and intervals

MPRs soft tissue	Slice thickness	Slice interval
Axial	3 mm	3 mm
Coronal (if required)	3 mm	3 mm
Sagittal	3 mm	3 mm

Computed tomography of cervical spine

MRI is now the preferred modality for assessing cervical discs and their interaction with the spinal cord. Trauma scans may however be performed along with head scans. In these instances DO NOT place the head in the head holder when a hard collar is in situ. Cervical spine scans, when they are used, extend from the skull base to T1, but patient size may dictate two ranges are performed to maintain image quality, especially if exposure modulation is not available and there is a need to reduce dose. If trauma type requires that a given area only is required to be scanned, some centres will use this option, then follow up with the trauma protocol to assess for neck stability at a later time.

Multislice scanning has enabled rapid scanning. This is especially useful in the unco-operative or severely injured patient and can be followed up with multiple MPRs (for these and cervical spine patients generally) by manipulation of the volume-acquired data set. Soft-tissue evaluation is best served by MRI. When MPRs are constructed they should be aligned with the vertebral bodies, and angled disc slices may also be generated. If 3D VR imaging is required, a thin overlapping data set using a soft-tissue algorithm is the best approach as this will create less noise than bone and hence enhance the images.

Spine: pathologies and indications

Pathologies		Indications	
	• cysts • disc and joint degeneration • disc herniation • fracture • spinal canal stenosis • tumours		• back/neck pain • paresthesia • sciatica • trauma

Cervical spine: WW and WL viewing values

Window	Width (HU)	Level (HU)
Bone	2000–3000	200–500
Soft tissue	150–450	30–50

Cervical spine: multislice spiral/helical protocol

Acquisition	No of detectors and width	Reconstruction thickness/ interval (mm)	mAs	kV	Algorithm	Rotation time	IV contrast
BOS–T1: axial helical	64 × 0.5 mm	1 mm/0.5 mm	~100 modulated	120	soft tissue and bone	0.5–1.0 second	X

Cervical spine: MPR planes, thickness and intervals, bone reconstructions

MPRs bone	Slice thickness	Slice interval
Axial	2 mm	2–3 mm
Coronal (if trauma)	2 mm	2–3 mm
Sagittal	2 mm	2–3 mm

Cervical spine: MPR planes, thickness and intervals, soft tissue reconstructions

MPRs bone	Slice thickness	Slice interval
Axial	3 mm	3 mm
Coronal	N/A	N/A
Sagittal	3 mm	3 mm

Computed Tomography Protocols

Computed tomography of thoracic spine

Trauma and metastatic spread are the primary reasons for CT of the thoracic spine, although IV contrast media is not always required to show spinal deposits; if unsure, check with the radiologist. A bone scan can be helpful in delineating the regions to scan in patients with known cancer. Positron emission tomography (PET) and CT are combined in a single machine to produce hybrid images that reveal physiological change linked to better-quality anatomical representation.

Correct vertebral level demonstration is essential so that the correct vertebra can be scanned from the pedicle above to the pedicle below the lesion. Sagittal MPRs accompany the axial images, and multiple planes can be reconstructed to demonstrate the extent and evaluate scoliosis. This ability is then used further in planning surgery, as pedicle size and scoliotic extent are necessary features for surgeons to evaluate. The ability to produce high-quality 3D VR representations has particular value in preoperative scoliosis cases.

Thoracic spine: WW and WL viewing values

Window	Width (HU)	Level (HU)
Bone	2000–3000	200–500
Soft tissue	150–450	30–50

Thoracic spine: multislice spiral/helical protocol

Acquisition	No of detectors and width	Reconstruction thickness/ interval (mm)	mAs	kV	Algorithm	Rotation time	IV contrast
C7–L1: axial helical	32 × 0.625 mm	1 mm/0.5 mm	–200	140	soft tissue and bone	0.5–1.0 second	X

Thoracic spine: MPR planes, thickness and intervals in bone

MPRs bone	Slice thickness	Slice interval
Axial	3–5 mm	3–5 mm
Coronal (if trauma)	3 mm	3–4 mm
Sagittal	3 mm	3–4 mm

Thoracic spine: MPR planes, thickness and intervals in soft tissue

MPRs soft tissue	Slice thickness	Slice interval
Axial	5 mm	5 mm
Coronal	N/A	N/A
Sagittal	3 mm	4 mm

Computed tomography of lumbar spine

MRI scans are the preferred method for showing lumbar disc (and spinal cord) lesions, though many CT examinations of this area still occur. Sciatic pain in lower back, hip and thigh are the main reasons to scan and if performed post myelogram (intrathecal injection of contrast medium) the patient should roll through 360° longitudinally on the scanner bed to spread the contrast evenly around the spinal cord. To prevent contrast migration and hence the risk of severe headaches due to contrast irritation of the meningeal spaces, scan the patient prone.

Trauma to the lumbar spine requires scanning as noted for thoracic spine. Identification of the correct vertebral level is again paramount. Sagittal MPRs should be generated with axial images. MPRs can also be generated for trauma or soft-tissue evaluation from a single volume acquisition. For disc examinations align the MPRs parallel with the vertebral body at that disc space.

Lumbar spine: WW and WL viewing values

Window	Width (HU)	Level (HU)
Bone	2000–3000	200–500
Soft tissue	150–450	30–50

Lumbar spine: multislice spiral/helical protocol

Acquisition	No of detectors and width	Reconstruction thickness/ interval (mm)	mAs	kV	Algorithm	Rotation time	IV contrast
(L1–S1) axial helical	64 × 0.5 mm	0.75 mm/0.5 mm	~300 modulated	140	soft tissue and bone	1.0 second	X

Lumbar spine: MPR planes, thickness and intervals in bone

MPRs bone	Slice thickness	Slice interval
Axial	0.75 mm	0.5 mm
Coronal (if trauma)	3 mm	3 mm
Sagittal	3 mm	3 mm

Lumbar spine: MPR planes, thickness and intervals in soft tissue

MPRs soft tissue	Slice thickness	Slice interval
Axial	0.75 mm	0.5 mm
Coronal	N/A	N/A
Sagittal	3 mm	4 mm

Computed tomography of sacrum and sacro-iliac joint

In an axial plane, carry out volume acquisition from S1 to the coccyx and generate MPRs in the sagittal, coronal and true axial planes.

Sacrum and sacro-iliac joint: WW and WL viewing values

Window	Width (HU)	Level (HU)
Bone	2000–3000	200–500
Soft tissue	150–450	30–50

Sacrum and sacro-iliac joint: multislice spiral/helical protocol

Acquisition	No of detectors and width	Reconstruction thickness/ interval (mm)	mAs	kV	Algorithm	Rotation time	IV contrast
L5 to end of coccyx: axial helical	16 × 1.5 mm	2 mm/1 mm	~280	140	soft tissue and bone	1.0 second	X

Sacrum and sacro-iliac joint: MPR planes, thickness and intervals in bone

MPRs bone	Slice thickness	Slice interval
Axial	3–5mm	3–5mm
Coronal (if trauma)	3mm	3–4mm
Sagittal	3mm	3–4mm

Sacrum and sacro-iliac joint: MPR planes, thickness and intervals in soft tissue

MPRs soft tissue	Slice thickness	Slice interval
Axial	5mm	5mm
Coronal	N/A	N/A
Sagittal	3mm	4mm

COMPUTED TOMOGRAPHY OF THORAX

Timing the acquisition correctly for thoracic imaging with intravenous contrast enhancement is crucial, and bolus tracking software should be employed. A good rule of thumb for timing related to cardiac output can be gleaned through cardiac shadow assessment on plain radiographs; a larger heart = longer time delay before arterial opacification. Apart from high-resolution lung parenchyma scans, IV contrast is indicated to aid the detection of mediastinal lymph node enlargement or vascular-related pathologies. The CT thoracic imaging IV contrast dose ranges across 75–120mL of 300–350 (300–370mg iodine per mL) strength contrast. Usually 1.5–2mL per kilogram (up to a total of 50mL) of 300mg/mL strength is sufficient in paediatric examinations.

Standard thoracic pathologies and indications

Pathologies	• abscess • contusion • haematoma • haemothorax • hiatus hernia • lymphoma • mesothelioma • neoplastic lesions • pericardial effusion • pneumothorax • septic emboli • teratoma • tuberculosis	Indications	• haemoptysis • mass on chest X-ray • shortness of breath

Chest: multislice spiral/helical protocol

Acquisition	No of detectors and width	Reconstruction thickness/ interval (mm)	mAs	kV	Algorithm	Rotation time	IV contrast
Axial helical	64 × 0.5 mm	2 mm/1 mm	~150	120	soft tissue and sharp/ lung	0.5–0.75 second	if required

Chest: MPR planes, thickness and intervals, soft tissue

MPRs soft tissue	Slice thickness	Slice interval
Axial	5–7 mm	5–7 mm
Coronal (if required)	5–7 mm	5–7 mm
Sagittal (if required)	5–7 mm	5–7 mm

Chest: MPR planes, thickness and intervals, lung

MPRs lung	Slice thickness	Slice interval
Axial	5–7 mm	5–7 mm
Coronal	5–7 mm	5–7 mm
Sagittal (if required)	5–7 mm	5–7 mm

Single short breath-hold acquisitions (e.g. 10 seconds) are possible, which reduces the chance of mis-registration artefacts and 'missed' data, so common in older scanner types. Thin-slice volume data sets are reconstructed into axial, coronal and sagittal MPRs with soft tissue and lung algorithms to enable nodule localisation, disease extent evaluation, pathology identification and airway analysis. Very thin lung slices are viewed in soft tissue and sharp or lung algorithms with thicker soft tissue and lung slices in the axial plane also being used. Using the data in thicker slabs, rather than creating MPRs in multiple planes (though coronal and/or sagittal MPRs are still created) enables vascular evaluation for pulmonary emboli identification or lung overview studies.

Thoracic pathologies and indications requiring HRCT

Pathologies	• bronchiectasis • fibrosis	Indications	• asthma • COAD • hypoxia

Chest/lung HRCT: sequence multislice protocol

Acquisition	No of detectors and width	Reconstruction thickness/ interval (mm)	mAs	kV	Algorithm	Rotation time	IV contrast
Axial sequence	2 × 1 mm	26 × 1 mm/ 10 mm	~200	140	soft tissue and sharp/lung	1.0 second	X

Chest/bronchiectasis HRCT: multislice spiral/helical protocol (CT angiography possible)

Acquisition	No of detectors and width	Reconstruction thickness/ interval (mm)	mAs	kV	Algorithm	Rotation Time	IV contrast
Axial helical	16 × 0.75 mm	1 mm/0.5 mm	~200	140	soft tissue and sharp/lung	0.5–0.75 second	if required

Computed Tomography Protocols

HRCT: MPR planes, thickness and intervals, soft tissue

MPRs soft tissue	Slice thickness	Slice interval
Axial	5–7 mm	5–7 mm
Coronal (if required)	5–7 mm	5–7 mm

HRCT: MPR planes, thickness and intervals, lung

MPRs lung	Slice thickness	Slice interval
Axial	1 mm	10 mm
Sagittal	5–7 mm	5–7 mm
Coronal	1 mm	10 mm

A helical or sequence multislice technique may be used to acquire high resolution CT (HRCT) of the lungs with pre-programmed techniques available as an option (i.e. differs from normal sequence approach) on multislice scanners where not all detectors have to be used. Volumetric data acquisitions collect sub-millimetre information that overlaps, so when 2D/3D software is applied MPRs of 1 mm thickness and 10 mm intervals in axial and coronal planes are possible. Thicker, contiguous (no gaps) data sets allow visualisation of the entire lung fields with coronal and axial MPRs created in lung and soft tissue viewing algorithms. If a routine chest CT plus HRCT is needed, both can be obtained simultaneously and, if acquired as an arterial data set, angiographic imaging is possible. This is advantageous in paediatrics where respiratory problems from congenital vascular or lung pathology impacts on the ability to secure high-quality images.

Chest/angiogram ?dissection: multislice spiral/helical protocol

Acquisition	No of detectors and width	Reconstruction thickness/ interval (mm)	mAs	kV	Algorithm	Rotation time	IV contrast
Axial helical	64 × 0.5 mm	2 mm/1 mm	~200	120	soft tissue	0.5–0.75 second	X
Axial helical	64 × 0.5 mm	1 mm/0.8 mm	~200 modulated	120	soft tissue and sharp/lung	0.5–0.75 second	✓

Aortic dissection: MPR planes, thickness and intervals, soft tissue reconstructions

MPRs + MIPS soft tissue	Slice thickness	Slice interval
Axial	2 mm	2 mm
Coronal	3 mm	3 mm
Sagittal aorta	3 mm	3 mm

Aortic dissection: MPR planes, thickness and intervals, lung reconstructions

MPRs lung	Slice thickness	Slice interval
Axial	3 mm	3 mm
Coronal	3 mm	3 mm

Thoracic dissection: WW and WL viewing values

Window	Width (HU)	Level (HU)
Soft tissue	300–700	30–70
Sharp lung parenchyma	800–1800	−300 to −700

Begin with a non-contrast acquisition from superior to the aortic arch to the aortic root to show calcification, as this may be obscured on a post-contrast scan. Use thin slices to minimise partial volume artefacts and enhance image quality for MPRs. Follow with a contrast scan (using thinner slices for greater resolution) in arterial phase from lung apices to the femoral fovea, as dissections may extend into iliac vessels. A further delayed scan of the second type can be performed to show pooling of contrast in the dissection flap. NOTE between 100 and 120 mL of 300–370 mg/mL at 3 or 4 mL/sec of iodinated contrast is used so there is potential renal impact. Use of a biphasic injection technique extends arterial temporal resolution and reduces contrast media. Dilution of IV contrast will reduce the hyperdense artefact commonly noted in the right brachiocephalic/superior vena cava. MPR, maximum intensity projections (MIPs) and VR images are constructed from the overlapping thin-slice volume data set.

CT pulmonary angiogram (CTPA): multislice spiral/helical protocol

Acquisition	No of detectors and width	Reconstruction thickness/ interval (mm)	mAs	kV	Algorithm	Rotation time	IV contrast
Axial helical	16 × 0.75 mm	1 mm/0.5 mm	~200	120	soft tissue and sharp/lung	0.5–0.75 second	✓

CTPA: MPR planes, thickness and intervals, soft tissue reconstructions

MPRs + MIPS soft tissue	Slice thickness	Slice interval
Axial	5 mm	5 mm
Coronal (if required)	5–10 mm	5 mm
Oblique	5–10 mm	5 mm

CTPA: MPR planes, thickness and intervals, lung reconstructions

MPRs lung	Slice thickness	Slice interval
Axial	5–7 mm	5–7 mm
Coronal	5–10 mm	5–10 mm

CTPA: WW and WL viewing values

Window	Width (HU)	Level (HU)
Soft tissue	300–700	30–70
Lung parenchyma	800–1800	−300 to −700

Due to faster scanning and bolus tracking software, the timing of scans and acquisition of thin-slice volumes has made contrast-enhanced images feasible in very short breath holds. Contrast should be injected at 4 mL/sec for CT pulmonary angiogram (CTPA). Thin overlapping data volumes can be reconstructed as MPRs in axial, coronal and curved oblique forms to be shown as thin and thick slices or slabs. Chest CT reconstructions can be achieved using the same data set (soft tissue and lung viewing algorithms) with axial and coronal MIPs to show the possible filling defects of pulmonary emboli. Due to the large number of images being generated and need to identify small emboli, the radiologist will review on screen and archive a representative sample of images for future reference.

Computed tomography of the heart

Cardiac CT angiography is performed for chest pain, previous myocardial infarction, coronary artery bypass grafts (CABG), family history of cardiac disease and hyperlipidaemia (raised blood fats). A vasodilator (sublingual, e.g. glyceryl trinitrate; GTN) is administered to ensure the 4th and 4th division arteries become visible, in conjunction with a beta blocker (if not con-traindicated) to decrease heart rate and extend the period during which images can be generated. This imaging approach is unsuit-able for patients with very high heart rates and sick sinus syn-drome (constantly changing heart rate).

A cardiac CT scan should include the whole of the heart extend-ing from the superior edge of the aortic arch to the diaphragm. The newest scanners of 256 and 320 slices can achieve a coronary artery image acquisition in a single rotation.

CT coronary angiogram: multislice spiral/helical protocol

Acquisition	Slice thickness	mAs	kV	Algorithm	Rotation time	IV contrast
Axial spiral, pitch 0.3–0.6	0.5–0.6 mm	300–500	120	soft tissue	0.3–0.4 sec	✓

CT coronary angiography: WW and WL viewing values

Window	Width (HU)	Level (HU)
Soft tissue range 1	400	100
Routine chest images	400	−1500 (large FOV)

Individual arteries (right and left main coronary, left descending, circumflex plus diagonal branches) are normally presented on a scan series. This is achieved by plotting along the curved vessel and demonstrating as a 2D image that can be rotated for examina-tion in multiple planes. A 3D VR image is normally included to show cardiac anatomy.

Chest, abdomen and pelvis: multislice spiral/helical protocol

Acquisition	No of detectors and width	Reconstruction thickness/ interval (mm)	mAs	kV	Algorithm	Rotation time	IV contrast
Chest: axial helical	16 × 1.5 mm	2 mm/1 mm (may do additional 7–10 mm recon)	~50–100	120	soft tissue and sharp/ lung	0.5–0.75 second	✓
Abdomen & pelvis: axial helical	16 × 1.5 mm	2 mm/1 mm (may do additional 7–10 mm recon)	~100–200	120	soft tissue	0.5–0.75 second	✓

Chest, abdomen and pelvis: MPR planes, thickness and intervals, soft tissue reconstructions

MPRs soft tissue (chest and abdomen)	Slice thickness	Slice interval
Axial (if not already reconstructed)	5–7 mm	5–7 mm
Coronal	5–7 mm	5–7 mm
Sagittal (if required)	5–7 mm	5–7 mm

Chest, abdomen and pelvis: MPR planes, thickness and intervals, lung reconstructions

MPRs lung	Slice thickness	Slice interval
Axial	5–7 mm	5–7 mm
Coronal	5–7 mm	5–7 mm
Sagittal (if required)	5–7 mm	5–7 mm

Due to fast acquisition speeds today, two data sets are required to show the chest, abdomen and pelvis (CAP). To show the portal venous phase of the abdomen and pelvic regions a delay is included, to prevent mismatching of scan acquisition with contrast media arrival to a region. The chest is scanned employing bolus tracking software or a built-in 30 sec delay which is followed by a further delay before the abdomen acquisition sequence begins at the top of the liver some 70 sec post injection. Delayed pelvic scans are not performed with routine studies, though trauma situations may dictate the need for further delay to show structures in the pelvic fossa. Use of an injection rate of 3 mL/sec enhances arterial opacification.

Volume-acquired thin overlapping data is used to create axial, coronal and occasionally thick-slice sagittal/oblique MPRs. Thin-sliced axial reconstructions are used to create the coronal and sagittal/oblique MPRs. Thick-slice axial slices are also reconstructed. For aortic angiographic studies (e.g. trauma, dissection) a single acquisition CAP is acquired in continuous arterial phase so the contrast enhancement of the aorta is sufficiently maintained to show all vessels clearly.

COMPUTED TOMOGRAPHY OF THE ABDOMEN

Due to the pathology specificity being linked to the protocol employed, abdominal CT scanning will need repeating if the incorrect approach is selected. Volume data acquisition allows post processing of thin slices through regions of interest when the patient has left the department.

IV contrast media is required for most abdominal protocols, with the timing of its administration being key to a successful examination; if timing is wrongly applied, post processing will not help. If calcifications are a component of the investigation, non-contrast scans should be performed initially as contrast will obscure detection of calcifications using abdominal windows and levels. Ensure suspended respiration during scanning as breathing causes organ blurring to suggest pathology is present.

Abdominal-pelvic pathologies and indications

Pathologies/Indications	<ul><li>abscess</li><li>aneurysm</li><li>appendicitis</li><li>ascites</li><li>bowel obstruction</li><li>Crohn's disease</li><li>diverticulitis</li><li>haemorrhage</li><li>hernias</li><li>ischaemic bowel</li><li>neoplasm</li><li>postsurgical collections</li></ul>

Abdomen and pelvis: multislice spiral/helical protocol

Acquisition	No of detectors and width	Reconstruction thickness/ interval (mm)	mAs	kV	Algorithm	Rotation time	IV contrast
Axial helical	64 × 0.5 mm	2 mm/1 mm (may do additional 7–10 mm reconstruction)	~100–200 modulated	120	soft tissue and sharp/ lung (lung bases)	0.5–0.75 second	✓

Abdomen and pelvis: MPR planes, thickness and intervals

MPRs soft tissue	Slice thickness	Slice interval
Axial (if additional reconstruction not done)	3 mm	3 mm
Coronal	3 mm	3 mm
Sagittal (if required)	3 mm	3 mm

Abdomen/pelvis (AP) scanning acquired volumetrically is used to generate thick and thin axial, coronal, sagittal and/or oblique MPRs. Thinner slices tend to be used for coronal and sagittal reconstructions. The whole acquisition can be obtained with a single breath-hold to reduce motion artefacts and this data set is used to also reconstruct further, thinner slices through regions of interest. Actually viewing the acquired thin slices is not necessary as they are reconstructed with increased spatial and contrast resolution as required. Further scan sequences will have to be obtained for differing contrast enhancement phases.

Renal pathologies and indications

Pathologies	• abscess • adenocarcinoma • angiomyolipoma • calcification • haemorrhage • hydronephrosis • lymphoma • polycystic renal disease • pyelonephritis • simple cysts • transitional cell carcinoma • urinoma	Indications	• haematuria • renal colic • renal transplant • trauma

General renal multislice spiral/helical protocol

Acquisition	No of detectors and width	Reconstruction thickness/ interval (mm)	mAs	kV	Algorithm	Rotation time	IV contrast
Range 1: axial helical, pitch 1.5	16 × 1.5 mm	2 mm/1 mm (may do additional 5 mm/5 mm)	~200–250	120	soft tissue adult body	0.5–0.75 second	X
Range 2: axial helical, pitch 1.5	16 × 0.75 mm	1 mm/0.5 mm (may do additional 5 mm/5 mm)	~200–250	120	soft tissue adult body	0.5–0.75 second	✓arterial
Range 3: axial helical, pitch 1.5	16 × 1.5 mm	2 mm/1 mm (may do additional 8 mm/8 mm)	~200–250	120	soft tissue adult body	0.5–0.75 second	✓venous

Renal: MPR planes, thickness and intervals

Arterial			Venous		
MPRs soft tissue	Slice thickness	Slice interval	MPRs soft tissue	Slice thickness	*Slice interval*
Axial (if additional reconstruction not done)	5 mm	5 mm	Axial (if additional reconstruction not done)	5–7 mm	5–7 mm
Coronal	5 mm	5 mm	Coronal	5–7 mm	5–7 mm
Sagittal (if required)	5 mm	5 mm	Sagittal (if required)	5–7 mm	5–7 mm

Renal colic (CT KUB): multislice spiral/helical protocol

Acquisition	No of detectors and width	Reconstruction thickness/ interval (mm)	mAs	kV	Algorithm	Rotation time	IV contrast
Range 1: axial helical	64 × 0.5 mm	2 mm/1 mm (may do additional 5 mm recon)	~100	120	soft tissue	0.5–0.75 second	X

Renal colic: MPR planes, thickness and intervals

MPRs soft tissue	Slice thickness	Slice interval
Axial (if additional reconstruction not done)	2.5–5mm	2.5–5mm
Coronal	2.5–5mm	2.5–5mm

Scan range 1: Scan non-contrast from superior to inferior poles of kidneys. Give a 50mL hand injection of IV contrast off the table and follow with a saline infusion of 500mL over 20 minutes. Further hydration by drinking water is also beneficial. Not all departments use the saline infusion and 20-minute delay technique, choosing to scan Range 2 and 3 after a 3-minute delay.

Scan range 2: Scan range 1 again in arterial phase employing an injection pump to deliver 70–100mL of IV contrast. Initiate the scan with tracking software or a delay of 20–30 seconds.

Scan range 3: Use the routine AP scan protocol to perform a venous phase scan between diaphragm and symphysis pubis with a 70-second delay from the start of the injection pump arterial delivery. Radiologists may prefer a 90-second delay to better show the kidney in its venous phase. The initial hand-injected 50mL of contrast and saline will by now have opacified the ureters and bladder for better visualisation, during the venous phase scan to reduce radiation dose. Although thinner slices will improve image quality, note that greater radiation dose (mAs increase) is required; though be sure the noise generation is sufficient to warrant this greater exposure.

Computed tomography of pancreas

Pancreas: pathologies and indications

Pathologies		Indications	
	• abscess • adenocarcinoma • islet cell tumour • pancreatitis (acute and chronic) • pseudocyst		• biliary duct dilatation • increased lipase • trauma

Pancreas: multislice spiral/helical protocol

Acquisition	No of detectors and width	Reconstruction thickness/ interval (mm)	mAs	kV	Algorithm	Rotation time	IV contrast
Range 1: axial helical, pitch 1.5	16 × 1.5 mm	2 mm/1 mm (may do additional 5 mm/5 mm)	~200–250	120	soft tissue adult body	0.5–0.75 second	X
Range 2: axial helical, pitch 1.5	16 × 0.75 mm	1 mm/0.5 mm (may do additional 5 mm/5 mm)	~200–250	120	soft tissue adult body	0.5–0.75 second	✓Arterial
Range 3: axial helical, pitch 1.5	16 × 1.5 mm	2 mm/1 mm (may do additional 8 mm/8 mm)	~200–250	120	soft tissue adult body	0.5–0.75 second	✓Venous

Pancreas: MPR planes, thickness and intervals

Arterial phase			Venous phase		
MPRs soft tissue	Slice thickness	Slice interval	MPRs soft tissue	Slice thickness	Slice interval
Axial (if additional reconstruction not done)	5 mm	5 mm	Axial (if additional reconstruction not done)	5–8 mm	5–8 mm
Coronal	5 mm	5 mm	Coronal	5–8 mm	5–8 mm
Sagittal (if required)	5 mm	5 mm	Sagittal (if required)	5–8 mm	5–8 mm

Scan range 1: Non-contrast scan between the superior and inferior pancreatic borders.

Scan range 2: Repeat range 1 in arterial phase (bolus tracking software or 20–30 sec post-injection delay using 100 mL volume at 3 mL/sec). This technique shows enhancement of the pancreatic parenchyma well and demonstrates necrotic changes in the pancreas to determine tissue death.

Scan range 3: Reviews the remaining upper abdominal region using the standard abdominal/pelvic protocol immediately tagged onto the pancreatic arterial phase acquisition.

Computed tomography of liver

Liver and spleen: pathologies and indications

Tumours (malignant)	Tumours (benign)	Other	Indications
• adenocarcinoma • cholangiocarcinoma • cirrhosis • gallbladder carcinoma • hepatoblastoma • hepatocellular carcinoma • lymphoma • metastases	• adenomas • focal nodular haemangioma • hamartomas • hyperplasia	• abscess • choledocholithiasis • cholelithiasis • cysts • fatty infiltration • hydatid • ruptured spleen • splenic infarct • subcapsular haematoma	• abnormal liver function tests • abnormality detected on ultrasound • hepatomegaly • jaundice • splenomegaly • trauma

Liver: multislice spiral/helical protocol

Acquisition	No of detectors and width	Reconstruction thickness/ interval (mm)	mAs	kV	Algorithm	Rotation time	IV contrast
Range 1: axial helical, pitch 1.5	16 × 1.5 mm	2 mm/1 mm (may do additional 5 mm/5 mm)	~200–250	120	soft tissue adult body	0.5–0.75 second	X
Range 2: axial helical, pitch 1.5	16 × 0.75 mm	1 mm/0.5 mm (may do additional 5 mm/5 mm)	~200–250	120	soft tissue adult body	0.5–0.75 second	✓ arterial
Range 3: axial helical, pitch 1.5	16 × 1.5 mm	2 mm/1 mm (may do additional 8 mm/8 mm)	~200–250	120	soft tissue adult body	0.5–0.75 second	✓venous

Multiphase liver: MPR planes, thickness and intervals

Arterial phase			Portal venous phase		
MPRs soft tissue	Slice thickness	Slice interval	MPRs soft tissue	Slice thickness	Slice interval
Axial (if additional reconstruction not done)	5 mm	5 mm	Axial (if additional reconstruction not done)	5–8 mm	5–8 mm
Coronal	5 mm	5 mm	Coronal	5–8 mm	5–8 mm
Sagittal (if required)	5 mm	5 mm	Sagittal (if required)	5–8 mm	5–8 mm

Scan range 1: Non-contrast superior to inferior borders of the liver (including the entire spleen). Repeat using bolus tracking software (aorta centred) or 20–30 sec after contrast to produce arterial phase images using 100 mL volume at 3 mL/sec.

Scan range 2: The portal venous phase scan is between the diaphragm and symphysis pubis. Sufficient delay is achieved (70 sec) in returning the table to the start position.

Scan range 3: Clinical indications or suspected pathology dictate the need for a further delayed phase; this repeats as the portal venous phase range.

Computed Tomography Protocols

The same detector configuration can be used for all phases, and the required thinner slices reconstructed through the region of interest from the data set. However, the detector combination can be adjusted for the arterial phase to enable higher resolution images (using thinner detector widths).

Clinical indications for CT of the adrenal glands

Tumours (malignant)	• adenomas • carcinoma • Cushing's syndrome • metastases • myelolipoma • phaeochromocytoma • primary aldosteronism • pseudotumours	Indications	• abnormal liver function tests • abnormality detected on ultrasound • hepatomegaly • splenomegaly • trauma

Adrenal glands: multislice spiral/helical protocol

Acquisition	No of detectors and width	Reconstruction thickness/interval (mm)	mAs	kV	Algorithm	Rotation time	IV contrast
Range 1: axial helical	16 × 1.5 mm	2 mm/1 mm (may do additional 8 mm/8 mm)	~200–250	120	soft tissue adult body	0.5–0.75 second	X
Range 2: axial helical	16 × 0.75 mm	1 mm/0.5 mm (may do additional 3 mm/3 mm through adrenals and 8 mm/8 mm through AP)	~200–250	120	soft tissue adult body	0.5–0.75 second	✓venous
Range 3: axial helical	16 × 1.5 mm	2 mm/1 mm (may do additional 3 mm/3 mm)	~200–250	120	soft tissue adult body	0.5–0.75 second	✓ 10 min delay

Adrenal glands venous phase: MPR planes, thickness and intervals

MPRs soft tissue	Slice thickness	Slice interval
Axial (if additional reconstruction not done)	3 mm	3 mm
Coronal	3 mm	3 mm
Sagittal (if required)	5 mm	5 mm

Scan range 1: Scan (non-contrast) from the superior to inferior borders of adrenals to determine the exact outline of the adrenal glands.

Scan range 2: Due to their small size, thinly collimated scans are employed through the adrenal glands post IV contrast in the portal venous phase. Use 100 mL contrast volume at 3 mL/sec.

Scan range 3: Follows the normal abdomen/pelvis range.

Scan range 4: Is used for adrenal lesion characterisation (adrenal washout). This scan is commenced 10 minutes after IV contrast administration begins, to enable adrenal lesion characterisation through washout features. Hounsfield unit measurements are taken through the adrenals at non-contrast, portal venous and delayed phases with the differing densities at each compared with tables to characterise a benign or malignant lesion.

Portal venous phase abdomen: MPR planes, thickness and intervals

MPRs soft tissue	Slice thickness	Slice interval
Axial (if additional reconstruction not done)	5–8 mm	5–8 mm
Coronal	5–8 mm	5–8 mm
Sagittal (if required)	5–8 mm	5–8 mm

Computed tomography: cholangiography

Investigation for choledocholithiasis (biliary stones in the duct and gallbladder) in the pre- or postcholecystectomy patient is the prime reason for the examination. The IV contrast medium used may be Biliscopin (meglumine iotroxate). Speed of introduction and contrast volumes are two key aspects of concern with this procedure. The following administration protocol is suggested (and see table below).

The patient fasts for 8 hours to ensure success of the CT cholangiogram. If the patient is in liver failure with a serum bilirubin level over 2.5 times normal (>50 µmol/L) then the examination could fail; 30 µmol/L is the limit in some departments.

The procedure is contraindicated for patients with hepatic and/or renal failure. A plain radiograph before the infusion is

commenced determines the presence of artefactual contrast
medium in the abdomen from previous procedures, as this may
hamper diagnosis. Procedurally, visualisation of contrast medium
in the duodenum signifies a successful examination. Air in the
biliary system can also be a contraindication unless it is present
post endoscopic retrograde cholangiopancreatography (ERCP),
as this may represent gas-forming organisms from an infective or
necrotic cause.

Biliscopin infusion protocol

Volume	100 mL Biliscopin
Patient position	Supine on a trolley
Starting infusion rate	10 mL over 10 minutes (60 mL/sec per hour) (check for any allergic reaction)
Finishing infusion rate (if no reaction)	90 mL over 20 minutes (270 mL/sec per hour)
Patient monitoring	15 minute blood pressure and pulse monitoring during infusion and 1 hour post examination
CT scan	Performed post infusion, best time is approx 45 mins

CT cholangiogram: WW and WL viewing values

Window	Width (HU)	Level (HU)
Soft tissue, range 1	300–700	50–150

Cholangiogram: multislice spiral/helical protocol

Acquisition	Slice thickness	Interval	mAs	kV	Algorithm	Rotation time	IV contrast
Range 1: axial spiral	5 mm		~100	120	soft tissue	0.5 second	✓
Range 2: axial spiral	0.5–2 mm		~150–250	120	soft tissue	0.5 second	✓
Reconstructions							
Sagittal cholangiogram	5	2.5			soft tissue		
Sagittal liver	5	5			soft tissue		
Coronal cholangiogram	5	2.5			soft tissue		
Coronal liver	5	5			soft tissue		

Range 1: A thick slice low radiation dose technique between T12 and L1/2 disc is employed to determine that the Biliscopin has been excreted by the liver. If Biliscopin is not present, repeat the scan 30–60 minutes post-infusion.

Range 2: When Biliscopin is present and has entered the duodenum then the patient can be scanned using the fine slice technique. The examination is acquired in suspended inspiration to cover the common bile duct and duodenal entry. Range suggested = diaphragm to iliac crest.

Computed tomography virtual colonography

CT virtual colonography (CTC) enables simultaneous viewing of the luminal mucosa of the colon and structures beyond the wall of the bowel. Appearances are similar to conventional colonoscopy, with CTC procedures designed to enable polyp differentiation from the mucosa using features such as virtual dissection and flythrough with reverse angle viewing. Polyps are seen clearly using lung windows on magnified axial slices, with structures beyond the colon being visualised with abdominal windows to see the abdominal and pelvic organs. MPRs are especially useful to evaluate the bowel wall perpendicular to the axial image, particularly at the flexures, transverse and sigmoid colon. Endoluminal 3D surface shaded (SS) and VR views add further detail to the images to differentiate polyps. CTC is advantageous where obstruction prevents conventional colonography progress or if the patient is unable to tolerate this invasive procedure, though biopsy and polyp removal is not possible and a large radiation dose is evident.

PATIENT PREPARATION AND DATA ACQUISITION

A 24 to 48 hour low-residue diet and the ingestion of a laxative for evacuation of colonic contents comprises appropriate imaging preparation. Faecal tagging = stool markers or iodine can also be administered orally 24 to 48 hours prior to CT; soft-tissue intraluminal lesions and retained faeces can therefore be differentiated. Any retained fluid is evacuated immediately before the scan and spasmolytic agents (Buscopan or glucagon depending on glaucoma status) are administered to reduce peristalsis and enhance distension during insufflations. Note the ileocaecal valve may be rendered patent so unwanted air refluxes into the small bowel. Where lesions need to be characterised, IV contrast agent can be administered but this is not required for screening purposes.

Room air or carbon dioxide is gently insufflated with the patient in the lateral decubitus position via a rectal catheter. Carbon dioxide has a steep diffusion gradient and is thought to decrease patients' discomfort from post-examination flatulence; obviously room air is readily available and cheaper. Usually 1.5 to 2 litres of air is required for good distension; a supine scout image is taken to confirm good distension with the catheter left in situ.

To perform CTC a dual positioning technique is used. Patients are initially scanned supine in a cephalocaudad direction covering the entire colon. The patient then turns prone with additional insufflations occurring at this time. A second scout localiser precedes the scan, which is repeated with a lower exposure over the same range. If prone positioning is impossible, scan the patient in the left lateral decubitus to optimise air and fluid redistribution. Dual positioning doubles the radiation dose but is required for optimal bowel distension and residual fluid redistribution to differentiate faeces from polyps. Filling defect motility signals retained faecal matter.

Continuous volume data sets are obtained with a single breath-hold (approximately 20 seconds) in supine and prone positions between the diaphragmatic domes and symphysis pubis. Slices are reconstructed between 1 mm and 5 mm thicknesses; thicker slices would miss smaller polyps.

CTC: multislice spiral/helical protocol

Acquisition	Detector configuration	Slice thickness	Interval	mA	kV	Algorithm	Rotation time	IV contrast
Range 1: supine axial spiral pitch 1.375:1	16 × 1.25	1.25 mm	0.6 mm	~60–160	120	soft tissue adult body	0.5 second	Not for screening
Range 2: prone axial spiral pitch 1.375:1	16 × 1.25	1.25 mm	0.6 mm	~60	120	soft tissue adult body	0.5 second	Not for screening

CTC: WW and WL viewing values

Windows	Width (HU)	Level (HU)
Lung-adjusted window settings	1200	200
Abdominal windows	350	50

Pelvimetry: single-slice sequence protocol on multislice scanner

Acquisition	Slice thickness	Table movement	mAs	kV	Algorithm	Rotation time	IV contrast
Axial sequence	10 mm	0 mm	~120–170	140	soft tissue adult body	1.5 second	X

Pelvimetry measurements

Measurement	Definition	Average value
AP outlet	From the inferoposterior border of the symphysis pubis, to the last fixed sacral segment	11.1 cm
Bispinous		10.4 cm
Inferior AP	From the mid-posterior border of the symphysis pubis through the ischial spine until the extended line meets the sacrum	11.8 cm
Superior AP	From the mid-posterior border of the symphysis pubis to the S3/S4 articulation	12.2 cm
Transverse		13.2 cm
True conjugate	From the superoposterior point of the symphysis pubis to the tip of the sacral prominence	11.4 cm

Computed Tomography Protocols

Lower thorax and whole abdomen: WW and WL viewing values

Window	Width (HU)	Level (HU)
Soft tissue abdomen range	300–500	30–60
Soft tissue liver parenchyma range	150–250	0–80
Soft tissue lung parenchyma range	800–1800	−300 to −700

COMPUTED TOMOGRAPHY OF EXTREMITIES

CT scanning of extremities is primarily used to demonstrate complex fractures and bony tumours. Intravenous contrast medium is rarely needed even in the investigation of neoplastic disease. Multiplanar reconstructions using varying viewing algorithms help ensure the maximum information is obtained from the scan. The bone algorithm is the most common method employed to reconstruct extremity scans. Sometimes, in the case of neoplastic disease or soft tissue injury, soft tissue images may also be created. In order to create 3D VR images, soft-tissue slice reconstruction is also performed.

Extremities: pathologies and indications

Pathology/Indication
• arthritis
• chondrosarcoma
• degenerative changes
• dislocation
• fibrosarcoma
• fracture
• giant cell tumour
• infections
• liposarcoma
• osteomyelitis
• osteonecrotic changes
• osteosarcoma
• postoperative evaluation

Positioning for CT imaging of extremities

Topogram	Examination	Patient positioning
Lateral topogram/ scout (to include joint under investigation)	axial foot/ankle coronal foot/ankle	• patient positioned supine, feet first • arms by patient's side or across chest • use Velcro straps and immobilisation pads to help the patient keep his/her feet/ankle still • use thick Velcro straps and strap the patient to the table for safety • ensure that patient is comfortable
AP topogram/ scout (to include entire joint under investigation)	axial wrist axial elbow sagittal wrist coronal wrist coronal elbow	• patient positioned prone, head first • arm to be investigated is placed above patient's head and rested on scan table • use Velcro straps and immobilisation pads to help the patient keep his/her arm still • use thick Velcro straps and strap the patient to the table for safety • ensure that patient is comfortable
AP topogram/ scout (to include entire shoulder joint)	axial shoulder	• patient positioned supine, head first • endeavour to get the shoulder to be imaged towards the isocentre of the gantry • affected arm by patient's side, other raised above head • use thick Velcro straps and strap the patient to the table for safety • ensure that patient is comfortable
AP topogram/ scout (to include joint under investigation)	axial knee axial acetabulum	• patient positioned supine, feet first • arms above patient's head • use thick Velcro straps and strap the patient to the table for safety • ensure that patient is comfortable • for knee examinations use sponge pads to keep the knee immobilised

Hand/wrist: multislice spiral/helical protocol

Acquisition	No of detectors and width	Reconstruction thickness/ interval (mm)	mAs	kV	Algorithm	Rotation time	IV contrast
Axial helical	32 × 0.625 mm	0.625 mm/0.3 mm	~60	120	bone (soft tissue if required)	0.75 second	X

Wrist: MPR planes, thickness and intervals

MPRs bone	Slice thickness	Slice interval
Axial	0.625 mm	0.625 mm
Coronal	0.5–1 mm	0.5–1 mm
Sagittal	0.5–1 mm	0.5–1 mm

This extremity protocol requires only a single acquisition and through use of true volumetric scanning enables the creation of MPRs in any plane without significant stair-stepping artefact.

Elbow: multislice spiral/helical protocol

Acquisition	No of detectors and width	Reconstruction thickness/ interval (mm)	mAs	kV	Algorithm	Rotation time	IV contrast
Axial helical	16 × 0.3 mm	1.5 mm/1.5 mm	~160	120	bone (and soft tissue if required and for 3D)	1.00 second	X

Elbow: MPR planes, thickness and intervals

MPRs soft tissue	Slice thickness	Slice interval
Axial	1.5 mm	1.5 mm
Coronal	1.5 mm	1.5 mm
Sagittal	1.5 mm	1.5 mm

Following trauma, the patient's elbow presents in an unwieldy position; scan with a volume data set with MPRs reconstructed from it in any plane to fully appreciate the extent of injury.

Shoulder: multislice spiral/helical protocol

Acquisition	No of detectors and width	Reconstruction thickness/ interval (mm)	mAs	kV	Algorithm	Rotation time	IV contrast
Axial helical	32 × 0.625 mm	0.625 mm/0.5 mm	~180	140	bone (soft tissue if required) and for 3D	0.75 second	X

Shoulder: MPR planes, thickness and intervals

MPRs bone	Slice thickness	Slice interval
Axial	1 mm	2 mm
Coronal	1 mm	2 mm
Sagittal	1 mm	2 mm

Sagittal and coronal MPRs +/− 3D VR from a multislice volume data set is the standard approach.

Foot/ankle: multislice spiral/helical protocol

Acquisition	No of detectors and width	Reconstruction thickness/ interval (mm)	mAs	kV	Algorithm	Rotation time	IV contrast
Axial helical	64 × 0.5 mm	0.5 mm/0.4 mm	~100	120	bone (soft tissue if required)	0.75 second	X

Foot/ankle: MPR planes, thickness and intervals

MPRs bone	Slice thickness	Slice interval
Axial	1 mm	2 mm
Coronal	1 mm	2 mm
Sagittal	1 mm	2 mm

This extremity protocol requires only a single acquisition and through use of true volumetric scanning enables the creation of MPRs in any plane without significant stair-stepping artefact. This reduces the importance of scanning in a direct axial or coronal plane though one should aim to position the patient correctly in one of these planes. Multislice is useful for patients unable to attain the correct position, for dose and image artefact reduction, and image quality issues. This technique enables sagittal MPRs, an image not normally available that can greatly assist the diagnosis of fractures and localisation. Patients in plaster casts are scanned in a single plane with reformations. As only a single scan is acquired, this may lead to a decrease in patient dose.

Knee: multislice spiral/helical protocol

Acquisition	No of detectors and width	Reconstruction thickness/ interval (mm)	mAs	kV	Algorithm	Rotation time	IV contrast
Axial helical	16 × 0.5 mm	0.5 mm/0.3 mm	~120	120	bone (soft tissue if required and for 3D)	0.75 second	X

Knee: MPR planes, thickness and intervals

MPRs soft tissue	Slice thickness	Slice interval
Axial	2 mm	2 mm
Coronal	2 mm	2 mm
Sagittal	2 mm	2 mm

Slightly thicker MPRs can be created, as the spatial resolution benefits of the 0.5 mm detector thickness are still present in the volumetric data set to generate the new thicknesses. MPR quality enables CT arthrogram studies of the knee to identify possible meniscal tears (when MRI is not possible), especially with bone and soft tissue reconstructions which may be necessary for this type of examination.

Hip/acetabulum: multislice spiral/helical protocol

Acquisition	No of detectors and width	Reconstruction thickness/ interval (mm)	mAs	kV	Algorithm	Rotation time	IV contrast
Axial helical	32 × 0.625 mm	0.625 mm/0.625 mm	~200 Auto mA	140	bone (soft tissue if required) and for 3D	0.5–0.75 second	X

Hip: MPR planes, thickness and intervals

MPRs (bone)	Slice thickness	Slice interval
Axial	1 mm	2 mm
Coronal	1 mm	2 mm
Sagittal	1 mm	2 mm

Excellent quality coronal and sagittal MPRs are achieved using multislice scanning techniques of the hip/acetabulum. Direct scanning of these planes is impossible but MPRs are very useful when visualising dislocated hips and fractures of the femoral neck or acetabulum. 3D VR imaging may also add value.

Further reading

Burdoff M. and Shinbone J. Eds (2006) *Cardiac CT Imaging: Diagnosis of Cardiovascular Disease*. Springer Verlag, London.

Dawson P.H. (2006) *Protocols for Multislice Helical Computed Tomography: The Fundamentals*. Taylor & Francis, London, New York.

Fishman E.K. and Jeffrey R.B. (Eds) (2003) *Multidetector CT: Principles, Techniques, and Clinical Applications*. Lippincott Williams & Wilkins, Philadelphia, PA.

Hofer M. (2005) *CT Teaching Manual: A Systematic Approach to CT Reading*. Thieme, Stuttgart.

Hosten N. and Liebig T. (2002) *CT of the Head and Spine*. Thieme, Stuttgart.

Prokop M. and Galanski M. (2003) *Spiral and Multislice: Computed Tomography of the Body*. Thieme, Germany.

Silverman P.M. (2002) *Multislice Computed Tomography: A Practical Approach to Clinical Protocols*. Lippincott, Williams & Wilkins, Philadelphia, PA.

Computed Tomography Protocols

Chapter 10

Magnetic Resonance Imaging Safety

Magnetic resonance imaging (MRI) uses a high field strength magnet, gradient fields and radio frequency fields to generate images. Standard MRI machine field strengths in use today are 1.5 T and 3 T (tesla) which poses problems in that some devices considered safe in the lower value magnet strength are not so in the higher strength unit. Some points to remember are as follows.

STATIC MAIN MAGNETIC FIELD

- Attracts and aligns magnetisable objects to the field – causes projectiles
- May apply torque and forces to implants and prostheses that could prove dangerous for patients
- As implants are possibly of various alloys, the magnetic effect on them is difficult to confirm

GRADIENT MAGNETIC FIELDS

- A current may be induced to stimulate the peripheral nervous system thus leading to reported phenomena by patients
- Acoustic noise is generated by the switching gradient field

Radio frequency (RF) safety issues

Due to the RF energy, nerve stimulation and heating may occur. This can be avoided by:

- Avoid looping of cables
- Use blankets and sheets etc. of materials such as cotton, linen, paper or dry material permeable to air

Index of Medical Imaging, First Edition. Jonathan McConnell.
© 2011 Blackwell Publishing Ltd. Published 2011 by Blackwell Publishing Ltd.

- Be sure the patient is not scanned in wet clothing or material dampened through perspiration
- Be sure the patient's hands, arms and legs do not touch and there is a 5mm gap between structures and tunnel wall covering
- Ensure adequate ventilation

Safety check for patients

Many departments operate a two-stage safety check for patients. This includes a preliminary check via the referrer, who is asked whether the patient has:

- A cardiac pacemaker
- A brain aneurysm clip
- An IVC filter
- A neuro stimulator
- A cochlear implant
- A Graseby (syringe) pump

If positive to any of these, then the scan may be refused.

When the patient arrives a full interview with safety check sheet should be performed to generate further details. **These first questions are employed to ascertain the likelihood of harm due to the interaction of the magnetic fields and RF impulses.** Typical questions would include:

Do you have:

- A cardiac pacemaker?   YES/NO
- A brain aneurysm clip?   YES/NO
- An inferior vena caval filter?   YES/NO
- A neuro stimulator?   YES/NO
- A cochlear implant?   YES/NO
- A Graseby (syringe) pump?   YES/NO

Where contrast agents may be used, ask:

- Hypertension?   YES/NO
- Diabetes?   YES/NO
- Kidney disease?   YES/NO
- Liver disease?   YES/NO

Do you have any allergies? YES/NO (if yes please detail these)	YES/NO
Have you ever had welding 'sparks' or metal in your eye?	YES/NO
If yes was this removed by a Doctor?	YES/NO
Are you pregnant?	YES/NO
What is your weight	___ kg

If you are aged over 60 please bring with you any recent blood test results.

Further questions that are related to heating risk, movement and therefore breakable implants and artefact generation are asked. Typically these include:

Do you have any of the following?

- Implanted heart valve
- Vascular heart clip or stent
- Carotid artery vascular clamp
- Embolisation coil
- Hickman's catheter
- PICC
- Brain shunt tube
- Hearing aid
- Ocular implant
- Joint replacement
- Metal pins or screws
- Harrington rod/spinal wires
- Wire sutures
- Intrauterine device
- Body jewellery
- Shrapnel, bullet or gunshot wound
- Dentures
- Inflatable breast implant
- Tissue expander
- Penile prosthesis
- Tattoos

Finally, before the patient consents to the use of contrast media, it is helpful to ascertain if the patient is claustrophobic or not as this will have impact on the performance of the scan.

Chapter 11

Magnetic Resonance Imaging Sequences

MRI Sequences

Musculoskeletal MRI examinations are generally performed to exclude a specific pathology or trauma that may be more difficult to delineate using other modalities. Not all examinations require IV contrast media. However, where there are suspicions of lesions that would be best visualised using a contrast agent, scans are sequenced with and without its use. MRI is used to define tumours, internal joint derangements, infections and subtle avascular necrosis of bones that may have been affected by trauma, possible infection or require evaluation of idiopathic cause. MRI is commonly used in specific bone or joint evaluation with the knee, shoulder, wrist, hip and spine being the most common examinations. The following suggestions are made for MRI examinations of these areas for specific reasons as indicated.

Index of Medical Imaging, First Edition. Jonathan McConnell.
© 2011 Blackwell Publishing Ltd. Published 2011 by Blackwell Publishing Ltd.

Musculoskeletal magnetic resonance imaging: knee

Internal derangement of knee joint

Plane	Acquisition	Area revealed
3 plane localiser		
Sagittal	FSE PD FSE T2	Meniscal lesion, ACL, PCL Meniscal lesion + fluid
Coronal	FSE T1 FSE T2 fat sat	Marrow, meniscal, ACL, PCL and collaterals Marrow, bone oedema, fluid
Axial	FSE PD	Patellar lesions, cartilage and ACL

Soft tissue tumour of knee

Plane	Acquisition
3 plane localiser	
Sagittal	FSE T2 fat sat FSE T1
Coronal	FSE T2 fat sat FSE T1
Axial	FSE T1 (PD if follow-up) FSE T2 fat sat
Contrast sagittal	FSE T1 fat sat
Contrast coronal	FSE T1 fat sat
Contrast axial	FSE T1 fat sat

Musculoskeletal magnetic resonance imaging: shoulder

Internal derangement of shoulder joint

Plane	Acquisition	Area revealed
3 plane localiser		
Oblique coronal	FSE T1 FSE T2 fat sat FSE PD	Marrow, supraspinatus Cuff tear, tendinopathy + fluid Cuff tear, superior labrum, supraspinatus
Oblique sagittal	FSE T2 fat sat PD	Cuff lesion and extent, bony oedema
Axial	PD fat sat	Labrum + subscapularis

MRI Sequences

Soft tissue tumour of shoulder

Plane	Acquisition
3 plane localiser	
Coronal	FSE T2 fat sat FSE T1
Axial	FSE T1 (PD if follow-up) FSE T2 fat sat
Contrast sagittal	FSE T1 fat sat
Contrast coronal	FSE T1 fat sat
Contrast axial	FSE T1 fat sat

Musculoskeletal magnetic resonance imaging: hip

Avascular necrosis and/or internal derangement of hip joint

Plane	Acquisition	Area revealed
3 plane localiser		
Coronal	FSE T1 both hips FSE T2 fat sat FSE PD	Marrow lesions Marrow oedema + joint effusion Labral tear
Axial	T2 fat sat PD fat sat	Lesion extent, bone oedema
Oblique sagittal	PD	Labral view

Arthrography/contrast media techniques

Arthrography protocol

Intra-articular	Indirect
• 20 gauge needle • 0.1 mL gadolinium in 25 mL saline • Inject until resistance felt, e.g. usually up to 20 mL for the knee	• IV gadolinium • 0.1 mmol gadolinium per kg bodyweight • Can be performed with or without exercise • No pre-contrast imaging • Injection 10–15 min prior to scan

Magnetic resonance imaging of the spine

Common investigations of the spine and spinal cord include evaluation for cord impingement, invasion by tumour or metastases, and establishing whether previous surgery has resulted in scar (granuloma) tissue that may cause pressure on the cord. Multiple sclerosis will reveal itself as characteristic plaques in spinal cord; therefore scanning is to include skull base through to conus. Mechanical causes for neuropathy can be ruled out using MRI as it is a very good modality for looking at soft tissues or those changes in bone tissue that occur following tumour, secondary deposits or infective invasion.

Myelopathy

Plane	Cervical spine	Lumbar spine
Localiser		
Sagittal	FSE T2 FSE T1	FSE T2 FSE T1
Axial	FSE T2 (through pathology)	FSE T2 (through pathology) FSE PD (through pathology)

Cervical spine degeneration

Plane	Acquisition
Localiser	
Sagittal	FSE T2 (small FOV, e.g. 24 cm) FSE T1
Axial	3D TOF GRE T2*

Cervical spine lesion

Plane	Acquisition
Localiser	
Sagittal	FSE T2 (larger FOV, e.g. 32–36 cm) FSE T1
Axial	FSE T2 (through lesion) FSE T1 (through lesion)

MRI Sequences

Cervical spine: syrinx

Plane	Acquisition
Localiser	
Sagittal	FSE T2 (larger FOV, e.g. 36 cm) FSE T1
Axial	FSE T2 (through lesion) FSE T1 (through lesion)
For first syrinx presentation also required are:	
Contrast sagittal	FSE T1
Contrast axial	FSE T1 (through lesion)

Cervical spine: multiple sclerosis plaques

Plane	Acquisition
Localiser	
Sagittal	FSE T2 FSE T1
Axial	FSE T2 (through pathology) FSE T1 (through pathology – optional)
Contrast sagittal	FSE T1 fat sat
Contrast axial	FSE T1 fat sat

Lumbar spine lesion

Plane	Acquisition
Localiser	
Sagittal	FSE T2 (larger FOV, e.g. 36 cm) FSE T1
Axial	FSE T2 (through lesion) FSE T1 (through lesion) No need for fat sat for T2 as marrow fat is used to provide contrast for the lesion

Lumbar disc prolapse

Plane	Acquisition
Localiser	
Sagittal	FSE T2 FSE T1
Axial	FSE T2 L3–S1 FSE PD L3–S1

Post spinal surgery

Plane	Acquisition
Localiser	
Sagittal	FSE T2 FSE T1
Axial	FSE T2 through surgery FSE PD through surgery
Contrast sagittal	FSE T1 fat sat
Contrast axial	FSE T1 fat sat

Spinal cord metastases

Plane	Cervical spine	Lumbar spine
Localiser		
Sagittal	FSE T2 FSE T1	FSE T2 FSE T1
Axial	FSE T2 (through pathology) FSE T1 (through pathology)	FSE T2 (through pathology) FSE T1 (through pathology)
Contrast sagittal	FSE T1 fat sat	FSE T1 fat sat
Contrast axial	FSE T1 fat sat	

Magnetic resonance imaging of the brain, head and neck

MRI's forte is in the soft tissue delineation of the brain. Previously, CT was the modality of choice in rendering the various soft tissue contrasts. Now MRI is able to give the best contrast and spatial resolution and demonstrate function in the brain using novel imaging techniques. Spectroscopy is adding to this ability and fusion of MRI and positron emission tomography (PET) images has added a great deal to spatial and functional representation. MRI is limited in use for trauma situations; however, longer-term evaluation, tumour rendition and visualisation of conditions such as multiple sclerosis have all been achieved with this imaging method. The soft tissue structures of the neck are clearly revealed to enable tumour and surgical staging of the pharyngeal areas, tongue and larynx.

Routine brain protocols

Plane	Stroke	Tumour (general)	Multiple sclerosis
Localiser			
Sagittal	FSE T1	FSE T1	FSE T1
Coronal			FLAIR (thin slices through corpus callosum)
Axial	FSE T2 FSE T1 FLAIR	FSE T2 FLAIR	FLAIR FSE T2 (whole brain + thin slices in posterior fossa)
Contrast sagittal			FSE T1 thin slices
Contrast coronal		FSE T1	
Contrast axial		FSE T1	FSE T1
Other sequences	DWI MRA Cor Grad	DWI	If contrast used need pre-contrast T1 Hi Res PF

General brain screening

Plane	Acquisition
Localiser	
Sagittal	FSE T2 (FOV 36 cm to cover whole cervicothoracic area) FSE T1
Axial	FSE T2 FLAIR
Optional sequences	DWI PD – can be gained in 1 scan using long TR + short & long TE to give PD & T2 in 1 sequence

Pituitary adenoma

Plane	Acquisition
Localiser	
Sagittal	T1
Coronal	FSE T1 (thin slices) FSE T2 (thin slices)
Axial	FSE T1 FSE T2 FLAIR
Contrast coronal	FSE T1 fat sat
Contrast axial	FSE T1
Optional sequences	+/– dynamic for micro tumours DWI Perfusion Spectroscopy

Cerebral abscess

Plane	Acquisition
Localiser	
Sagittal	FSE T1
Coronal	FSE T2 fat sat (thin slices)
Axial	FLAIR
Contrast sagittal	FSE T1 (thin slices)
Contrast coronal	FSE T1 (thin slices)

Trauma

Plane	Acquisition
Localiser	
Sagittal	FSE T1
Coronal	Cor Grad Echo
Axial	FSE T2 FSE T1 FLAIR

MRI Sequences

The auditory system

Plane	Acquisition: internal auditory meatus	Acquisition: acoustic neuroma
Localiser		
Coronal	SSFSE 3D thin slices	
Axial	SSFSE 3D thin slices FSE T2 (whole brain)	SSFSE 3D thin slices FSE T1
Contrast coronal		FSE T1
Contrast axial		FSE T1

Magnetic resonance imaging of the abdomen

MRI imaging of the abdomen has some problems associated with it related to an inability to prevent bowel movement (or to scan in a short enough acquisition time) such that artefacts termed ghosting, blurring and that due to bowel movement are often registered. If a patient is unco-operative this may lead to further difficulties. Patients are usually fed into the scanner feet first and a torso coil is used in adults. Children by comparison may be small enough to fit within a head coil. With longer scan times, headphones are useful to provide distraction and noise suppression and to maintain patient contact, with compression band use also aiding the reduction of involuntary movement.

Liver

Plane	Acquisition
Localiser	
Axial	FSE T2 f/s gated GRE T1 breath-hold GRE T2 breath-hold
Contrast coronal	High res T1 breath-hold
Contrast axial	Dynamic GRE T1 fat sat High res T1 breath-hold

MRI Sequences

Pancreas

Plane	Acquisition
Localiser	
Axial	FSE T2 f/s gated GRE T1 breath-hold GRE T2 breath-hold
Contrast coronal	High res T1 thin breath-hold
Contrast axial	Dynamic GRE thin T1 fat sat (2mm slices) High res T1 thin breath-hold

Magnetic resonance cholangiopancreatography

Plane	Acquisition
Localiser	
Axial	FSE T2 FSE T1 High res T1 f/s
Coronal	STIR
Other sequences	Dynamic T1 f/s GRE

Chapter 12

Typical Effective Doses from Diagnostic Medical Imaging Procedures

The Royal College of Radiologists (United Kingdom) indicates that whole-body background radiation received in the UK varies between 1.5 and 7.5 mSv per year according to regional variation, though it is suggested that 2.2 mSv is a more usual average value. In the United States the Health Physics Society has indicated the average background dose received by most Americans is closer to 3.0 mSv.

In line with the RCR's idea of relating dose to numbers of chest images or comparing against days of typical background dose, the following is suggested as the likely dose received for medical diagnostic procedures listed below. (The figures are from the United States, which are higher than those in the UK, but equate to practices in many other countries.)

Index of Medical Imaging, First Edition. Jonathan McConnell.
© 2011 Blackwell Publishing Ltd. Published 2011 by Blackwell Publishing Ltd.

Procedure	Typical effective dose (mSv)	Equivalent chest X-rays (PA + Lat)	Background equivalence
Radiography			
Chest (PA + Lat)	0.1	1	15 days
Chest (PA only)	0.02	0.2	3 days
Thoracic spine	1.0	10	5 months
Lumbar spine	1.5	15	7 months
Pelvis	0.7	7	4 months
Abdomen or hip	0.6	6	4 months
Mammogram (two-view)	0.36	3.6	55 days
Dental (OPG)	0.01	0.1	2 days
DEXA (whole body)	0.001	0.01	0.2 days
Skull	0.08	0.8	12 days
Limb	<0.01	0.1	2 days
Contrast studies/CT			
IVU	3.0	30	16 months
Barium swallow	1.5	15	8 months
Barium meal + FT	6.0	60	32 months
Barium enema	7.0	70	3 years
CT head	2.0	20	10 months
CT chest	7.0	70	3 years
CT abdomen/pelvis	10	100	4.5 years
CT biopsy	1.0	10	5 months
CT Ca^{2+} scoring	2.0	20	10 months
Radionuclide			
Lung Q/V	2.5	25	1 year
Bone	6.3	63	33 months

(*Continued*)

Medical Imaging Procedures

Procedure	Typical effective dose (mSv)	Equivalent chest X-rays (PA + Lat)	Background equivalence
Heart tests (various)	9.4–41.0	94–410	4–17 years
Brain	14.1	141	6 years
Tumour/Infection	2.5	25	1 year
Hepatobiliary studies	2.1	21	11 months
Kidney (various)	1.8–2.2	18–22	9–11 months
Vascular – DSA			
Coronary angiogram	20	200	9 years
Coronary + intervention	30	300	13.5 years
Pacemaker placement	1.0	10	5 months
Peripheral + plasty	5.0	50	2 years

Source: Health Physics Society (January 2010) *Radiation Exposures from Medical Exams and Procedures*. McLean, VA, USA. Available at http://hps.org/documents/Medical_Exposures_Fact_Sheet.pdf (accessed 26 August 2010).

Medical Imaging Procedures

Chapter 13

Indicated Imaging

INDICATED EXAMINATIONS FOR THE DIAGNOSIS OF COMMON TRAUMA PRESENTATIONS

Indication	Order and investigation type (relative radiation level)	Comments
Cervical spine		
Patient conscious and has head or face only injury	1. Cervical spine X-ray (1) 3 views normal – CT required if technically inadequate imaging	Associated risk factors indicating need for cervical spine radiography: <45° neck rotation; <15 GCS; 65 yrs or over; focal neurological deficit or extremity parasthesia; mechanism of injury, e.g. fall over 1 m; injury not of following nature so unable to assess safely: simple rear-end impact; walking since injury; delayed neck pain onset; sitting in A&E; no midline cervical spine tenderness.

(*Continued*)

Index of Medical Imaging, First Edition. Jonathan McConnell.
© 2011 Blackwell Publishing Ltd. Published 2011 by Blackwell Publishing Ltd.

Indication	Order and investigation type (relative radiation level)	Comments
Patient unconscious with head injury	1. CT (primarily) (2) 2. Cervical spine X-ray (1)	Diagnostically adequate cervical spine X-rays are difficult to achieve in unconscious patients. In high-risk injuries CT of whole cervical and upper thoracic spine indicated.
Painful neck injury	1. Cervical spine X-ray (1) 2. CT (2) 3. MRI (0)	Factors indicated as for the head or facially injured conscious patient. CT is appropriate for high-risk or complex injuries or equivocal findings on X-ray. MRI has a role for complex cases, especially soft tissue injuries.
Neurological deficit neck injury	1. Cervical spine X-ray (1) 2. MRI (0) 3. CT (2)	Cervical spine X-ray acts as baseline orthopaedic assessment and for surgical planning. Intrinsic cord damage and compression +/– ligament injury and multiple level fractures are best revealed by MRI. CT cervical spine when good-quality radiography not possible. CT myelography an alternative when unable to provide MRI.

Indicated Imaging

Indication	Order and investigation type (relative radiation level)	Comments
Cervical spine		
Possible ligamentous neck injury	1. Cervical spine X-ray (1) 2. MRI (0)	Flexion and extension views may be used 10+ days post-injury only if possible with no assistance and under medical supervision. MRI of greater value in the acute context.
Thoracolumbar spine		
Trauma – no pain or neuro deficit	1. Radiograph (1)	Even though a possible examination, physical evaluation should be relied upon when patient is alert, asymptomatic and no neurology. Radiological findings rarely change management.
Trauma – pain, no neuro deficit or unable to evaluate patient	1. Radiograph (1)	Radiographic correlation with injury is good with pain or tenderness following high falls or high-energy road accidents or if another spine fracture evident. Good overview achievable for low dose if unable to evaluate patient. Radiographic signs of instability should have supporting CT or MRI performed.

Indicated Imaging

(*Continued*)

Indication	Order and investigation type (relative radiation level)	Comments
Thoracolumbar spine		
Trauma – with neuro deficit +/– pain	1. Radiograph (1) 2. CT (2) 3. MRI (0)	Radiography is used as an initial investigation. CT and MRI should accompany to give good bone rendition (CT) or when multiple level problems +/– ligament or cauda equina injuries (MRI).
Pelvis and sacrum		
Fall – unable to bear weight	1. Pelvis + lateral hip X-ray (1)	Not all fractures show, even on good images. With less successful clinical exams consider Nuclear Medicine, MRI or CT if radiography equivocal.
Pelvic injury + bleeding from urethra	1. Retrograde urethrogram (2)	Used to show if a leak, tear or integrity of urethra in doubt. Consider delayed post-contrast CT to assess for other urinary injuries if haematuria and urethra normal. MRI could be used in non-urgent situations.
Coccydinia or trauma to coccyx	1. Radiograph (1)	Value of radiography limited as normal appearances easily confused as abnormal and vice versa; limited management impact even if injury identified.

Indicated Imaging

Indication	Order and investigation type (relative radiation level)	Comments
Upper limb		
Wrist +/– scaphoid fracture	1. Radiograph (1) 2. MRI (0) 3. NM (2) 4. CT (2)	A four view series is required for scaphoid fracture exclusion – otherwise a minimum of 2 projections for wrist. MRI now used as a first-stage exam to identify scaphoid injury. Any of the modalities may be used to identify, though MRI is now preferable (and often the only further modality) due to its better specificity.
Elbow trauma	1. Radiograph (1)	Radiography clearly reveals effusion and without this routine follow-up examinations are not suggested. MRI may be used in the most difficult cases.
Shoulder trauma	1. Radiograph (1)	At least orthogonal views are necessary as some findings are subtle in nature. US, MRI and CT have a role in evaluating complex soft tissue injuries. Rotator cuff damage should be considered in the 50+ age group where poor mobilisation follows a 1st dislocation.

Indicated Imaging

(*Continued*)

Indication	Order and investigation type (relative radiation level)	Comments
Lower limb		
Foot injury	1. Radiograph (1)	Bone tenderness and inability to bear weight are the key indicators. Complex hindfoot injuries should be evaluated with CT, forefoot injury demonstration rarely affects management. Foot and ankle as a request rarely shows injury of both – refer Ottawa guidelines; good reasons required for both to be obtained.
Ankle injury	1. Radiograph (1) 2. US (0) 3. MRI (0) 4. CT (2)	Ottawa rules that justify radiography are: non-weight-bear immediately and in A&E; tender over any posterior malleolar edges. US, MRI and CT are used to show soft tissue and occult bone injuries. radiologist advice required.
Knee trauma due to blunt injury/fall	1. Radiograph (1)	Radiography clearly indicated when fall/blunt trauma mechanism in <12 or >50 or unable to bear weight for 4 steps. If further info required by imaging CT = intra-articular fracture, MRI = ligament or meniscal injury, US = extensor mechanism injury.

Indication	Order and investigation type (relative radiation level)	Comments
Stress fracture	1. Radiograph (1) 2. NM (2) 3. MRI (0) 4. CT (2)	Often minimal results though radiography is appropriate. Helpful for early detection due to use of physiological properties impacted upon by injury. US is being used in some instances.
Chest		
Minor chest trauma	1. Radiograph (1)	Will result in no change of management when CXR performed for possible rib fracture. Good selection if complication such as pneumothorax suspected.
Stable patient with moderate chest trauma	1. Radiograph (1) 2. CT	Erect CXR required to exclude pneumothorax or show pleural fluid or differentiate from lung contusion. If aortic trauma suspected CT appropriate and will reveal pneumothorax not visible on plain radiograph.
Stabbing	1. Radiograph (1)	Standard PA +/− other projections will show lung damage, fluid or pneumothorax. CT or US are helpful to show pericardial and pleural fluid collections.

(*Continued*)

Indication	Order and investigation type (relative radiation level)	Comments
Sternal injury	1. Radiograph (1)	Lateral sternum + chest radiograph are obtained to show injury – thoracic spine and/or aortic injuries should also be considered thus requiring a full lateral chest image.
Abdomen		
Blunt or stab injury	1. Chest radiograph (erect) (1) Abdomen radiograph (supine) (1) 2. US (0) 3. CT (3)	Some centres continue to request an erect abdomen when the erect chest and supine abdomen will reveal most information for minimal radiation. Ultrasound will detect some injuries/ haematomata to organs such as liver and spleen. A high dose specialised examination – consult radiologist.
Kidney trauma	1. CT (3) 2. Contrast radiography (2) 3. US (0)	CT reveals most information in renal trauma following major injury +/– hypotension +/– frank haematuria. Delayed contrast (excretion phase) CT should be included to assess the renal collecting system. IVU is useful in adults with blunt kidney trauma and no other features as above – CT can be avoided in these cases. Ultrasound helpful in initial assessment but negative US does not exclude renal injury.

Indication	Order and investigation type (relative radiation level)	Comments
Foreign body detection		
ST injury + FB of metal, glass painted wood	1. Radiograph (1) 2. US (0)	As long as blood-stained dressings are removed, glass which is radio-opaque should be visible. If the FB is radiolucent or X-ray uncertain then US may have a role.
ST injury + FB of plastic, wood	1. Radiograph (1) 2. US (0)	Plastic and wood rarely show on radiographs. US is more likely to reveal FBs that are invisible radiographically.
Ingested FB – pharynx or upper oesophagus	1. Radiography – neck Neck + chest in paediatrics (1) 2. Radiography – abdomen (1)	Only use radiography post oropharyngeal examination (as probably lodged there) and if the FB is radio-opaque. Ca^{2+} in cartilage makes differentiation difficult – most fish bones are radiographically invisible. Bronchoscopy is mandatory for inhaled FB in paediatrics. Consider fluoroscopy to view air trapping which may be difficult to confirm on expiration chest image. Of value only if radio-opaque or likely to have signs of obstruction. If still pain or greater suspicion consider laryngoscopy or endoscopy. Failure to pass after 6 days by paediatrics should prompt an abdominal radio-graph, as should swallowing of sharp or possibly poisonous FBs, e.g. batteries.

Indicated Imaging

(*Continued*)

Indication	Order and investigation type (relative radiation level)	Comments
Smooth, small ingested FB	1. Radiograph – chest (1) 1. Radiograph – abdomen (1)	Paediatrics should have neck and chest images and adults may also require a lateral chest for localisation; however FBs are rarely radio-opaque. As most FBs impact at the cricopharyngeal narrowing, the chest image will be sufficient. If definitely known to be abdominal then failure to pass after 6 days should prompt abdominal X-ray localisation.
Sharp or maybe poisonous ingested FB	1. Radiograph – abdomen (1) 1. Radiograph – chest (1)	Usually if a swallowed FB clears the oesophagus then it will move through the GI tract; items that may be poisonous, e.g. batteries, should be localised in case of leakage. If the abdominal image is negative a chest radiograph should be obtained.

Indication	Order and investigation type (relative radiation level)	Comments
Craniofacial trauma		
Head injury: brain injury risk is high when: GCS ≤ 12 since trauma	1. CT (2) 2. MRI (0) 1. Radiograph – skull (1)	With head injury patients CT should be available to evaluate fully and take place within local protocol. If memory loss or significant injury mechanism with no other brain injury characteristics, CT may be delayed. GCS ↓ during observation requires early CT performance; a persistent reduced GCS at 24 hrs suggests repeat CT or MRI investigation. If any new lesions are evident on the CT of a head injured patient, if CT is not available or clinically a neurosurgical intervention (including assessment and monitoring) is suggested then consult neurosurgery. MRI should be employed in trauma situations as outlined above. Skull radiography has limited use and in cases other than triage if CT is unavailable or as a constituent of the skeletal survey of paediatrics. In the 0–2 yr skeletal survey patient a head CT is mandatory.
GCS = 13/14 at 2+ hrs post trauma		
Open or depressed skull fracture		
? Skull base fracture		
1+ x vomiting post trauma		
Seizure, new or evolving focal neurology post injury		
65+ yrs or coagulopathy + amnesia or ↓ consciousness		

(*Continued*)

Indication	Order and investigation type (relative radiation level)	Comments
Craniofacial trauma		
Nose trauma	1. Radiograph (1)	As X-rays are diagnostically unreliable and add nothing to management of nasal trauma, they only have a role in follow up ENT/maxillofacial treatment.
Orbital injuries – blunt	1. Radiograph – facial bones (1)	X-rays should be used with suspicion of blowout fracture. If clinical and radiographic signs are equivocal or persistent diplopia then MRI or direct coronal CT could be adjunctive imaging.
Orbital injuries – penetrating	1. Radiograph – orbits (1) 2. CT (2) 3. US (0) 4. MRI (0)	X-rays are very helpful to identify retained metallic intraorbital FBs. If radio-opacity of suspected FB is low, e.g. nonmetal or small size, then CT is helpful. Anterior intraocular FBs can be detected using US. MRI and metallic FBs are a hazardous combination! Where strong clinical suspicion persists and other imaging does not reveal an FB specialised investigation may be performed.

Indicated Imaging

Indication	Order and investigation type (relative radiation level)	Comments
Facial injury – mid 1/3	1. Radiograph – facial bones (1) 2. CT (2)	Radiography has limited use due to the 3D nature of fracture tracking – low dose CT for complex injuries is an option though patient co-operation requirements are high, thus indicating a delay until achievable.
Mandible trauma	1. Radiograph – mandible (1) 2. OPG (1)	As the equipment requires the patient to be erect an OPG will not be feasible on the multiply injured patient. Several radiographic projections will provide an equivalent outcome.
Major trauma		
Screen of the unconscious or confused patient	1. Radiograph – CXR (1) 1. Cervical spine (1) 1. Pelvis (1) 2. CT (2)	Only initial assessment images should be obtained until stabilisation of the patient is achieved. This may mean CXR and pelvis take precedence over the appropriately protected cervical spine due to haemodynamic and ventilatory concerns. If CT of head or body is anticipated the cervical spine may also be included thus negating the need for plain radiographs.

(*Continued*)

Indicated Imaging

Indication	Order and investigation type (relative radiation level)	Comments
Major trauma to chest, abdomen and pelvis	1. Radiograph – CXR (1) 1. Pelvis (1) 2. US (0) 3. CT (3)	(Haemo/hydro) pneumothoraces should be excluded and other significant signs visible on the CXR should be accounted for. Pelvis radiography is required as pelvic ring disruption is associated with major blood loss. US is used in resuscitation to show free fluid or solid organ injury but has low sensitivity for spleen GI and urinary tract injury. Peritoneal lavage is a further option. Sensitivity and specificity of CT makes it the investigation of choice and could negate the need for plain radiography and US if appropriate image reconstruction techniques are available. Mediastinal haemorrhage/aortic injury are strong points of multidetector CT techniques.

INDICATED EXAMINATIONS FOR THE DIAGNOSIS OF COMMON MUSCULOSKELETAL PRESENTATIONS

Indication	Order and investigation type (relative radiation level)	Comments
Spine		
Degenerative neck pain +/– arm involvement	1. Cervical spine X-ray (1) 2. MRI (0)	Conservative management often results in pain resolution – although degenerative changes are evident on images there may not often a symptom link. MRI should be employed if suspicion of neurology or when pain affects lifestyle. Consider CT myelography if MRI unavailable or further information required.
Possible C1/C2 subluxation	1. Cervical spine X-ray (1) 2. MRI (0) 3. CT (2)	Use a single lateral cervical image with flexion under supervision to reveal significant changes in the rheumatoid arthritis patient or those with trisomy 21. MRI will reveal spinal cord involvement after and is used following +ve X-ray or with neurological signs. Congenital and structural problems (leading to subluxation) are best revealed by CT. Rotational subluxation following trauma is also best revealed using this modality.

(*Continued*)

Indicated Imaging

Indication	Order and investigation type (relative radiation level)	Comments
Spine		
Atraumatic nondegenerative thoracic spine pain	1. MRI (0) 2. Thoracic spine X-ray (1)	MRI is helpful in persistent local pain or when management is difficult. It should also be employed with long tract signs (voluntary motor function, pain, temperature, crude touch and proprioception) are evident. Degenerative changes are commonly visible from middle age onwards. Thoracic spine radiography is most helpful when neurology is present or indication of metastatic or infective diseases. Osteoporotic collapse (or other bone collapse causes) in the aged will deliver sudden pain. Consider NM for metastases.
Chronic lumbar spine pain with no infective or neoplastic indicators	1. MRI (0) 2. Lumbar spine X-ray (1) 3. CT (2) 4. Nuclear Med (2)	MRI is the examination of choice for spinal diseases. Radiography should be performed with collapsed vertebral investigation (osteoporosis/metastases) or spondyloarthropathy in younger patients. If MRI is contraindicated use CT or for further bone assessment, e.g. spondylolysis. NM may show hidden spondylolysis or tumours such as osteoid osteoma. MRI and CT are preferential due to increased specificity.

Indication	Order and investigation type (relative radiation level)	Comments
Acute back pain with serious indicators, e.g. widespread neurological deficit or progressive motor loss; saddle numbness; sphincter and gait disturbance; <20 or >55; previous cancer; HIV; wt loss; IV drug user; fever; thoracic pain; spinal deformity; -ve pain relief with bed rest; systemic illness	1. MRI (0) 2. Radiography (1) 3. CT (2) 4. Nuclear Med (2)	Perform MRI immediately with those presenting neurological features and urgently if suspicion of malignant or infective disease. A useful preoperative investigation but MRI will give a better negative prediction of disease presence. Use CT in biopsy of bone or soft tissue. It will also show sequestra as a result of infections. NM best shows full extent of disease (e.g. metastases) and should be used in conjunction with plain radiography.
Acute back pain minus serious indicators	1. MRI (0) 2. CT (2) 3. Radiography (1)	MRI reveals a larger area of interest so is the preferred method. Disc herniation after conservative treatment should be considered but needs clinico-radiological correlation as asymptomatic herniation is frequent. Radiography rarely demonstrates diseases on images (other than porotic collapse) and so reassures inappropriately.

(Continued)

Indication	Order and investigation type (relative radiation level)	Comments
Bone conditions		
Osteomyelitis	1. Radiography (1) 2. MRI (0) 3. US (0) 4. CT (2) 5. Nuclear Med (2)	Radiography should be performed initially with MRI being most accurate at revealing bone and soft tissue changes linked with osteomyelitis. Consider MRI as the best technique in suspected cases. US may show subperiosteal collections/abscesses but is less sensitive than MRI. CT is best used to demonstrate sequestra and to localise for biopsy. NM may be used with Tc-99-HMPAO or In-111 white cell labelled techniques. Skeletal scans may help localise but results are nonspecific to osteomyelitis. If periprosthetic infection suspected, NM is helpful. PET can be used in chronic osteomyelitic situations.
Primary bone tumour	1. Radiography (1) 2. MRI (0) 3. Nuclear Med (2) 4. US (0) 5. CT (2)	X-ray is the first examination to investigate failure to resolve bone pain. If results are suggestive of primary tumour, MRI should be used to stage, preferably at a specialist centre. NM skeletal nuclear medicine to exclude multiple deposits should occur. FDG-PET may have a role. If tumour is relatively superficial in the tissue, US may be used to guide a biopsy. CT can be used to better characterise tumour patterns. It too may be used in biopsy guidance; in both biopsy situations specialist histological and surgical support should be enrolled.

Indication	Order and investigation type (relative radiation level)	Comments
Skeletal secondaries	1. MRI (0) 2. Nuclear Med (2) 3. Skeletal survey X-ray (2)	MRI is the best technique re sensitivity and specificity compared with NM. May undervalue peripheral skeletal lesions. If a known primary cancer then NM good for detection of secondaries but will not delineate myeloma. Correlating images improve NM specificity. NM may be applied to assess treatment response but should only be used 6/12 after treatment or less if new symptoms appear. X-rays improve NM specificity or add information to localised areas displaying symptoms.
Bone pain	1. Radiography (1) 2. MRI (0) 3. Nuclear Med (2) 4. CT (2)	Dedicated views of the area under suspicion can be provided though may be of limited value at times. MRI should be used with persistent pain + normal X-ray or NM. Further findings may be given by MRI in abnormal X-ray and NM examinations. Diffuse bone pain is less able to be evaluated with MRI. If pain persistent with normal or uncertain X-ray results NM should be used. With abnormal X-ray NM help characterise, e.g. second-aries, osteomyelitis or specific tumours such as osteoid osteoma. Bone anatomy is clearly defined by CT where abnormal examinations of other modalities have been obtained. This feature is particularly helpful should bone biopsy be required.

Indicated Imaging

(*Continued*)

Indication	Order and investigation type (relative radiation level)	Comments
Myeloma	1. Skeletal survey X-ray (2) 2. MRI (0) 3. Nuclear Med (2)	X-ray sensitivity is good in the pelvis, spine and upper femurs. Follow-up examinations and tumour mass evaluation is also well served by plain X-ray. If patient is osteopenic or myeloma non-secretory in nature (2% of cases), X-ray also provides good imagery. MRI is best used in identification of lesions for radio-therapeutic treatment and follow-up evaluation. MRI can be limited to specific areas/lesions in follow-up procedures. Skeletal NM is commonly negative for myeloma or at least underestimates the extent of the disease. Bone marrow studies may add in these instances.
Metabolic bone diseases	1. Radiography (2) 2. DEXA (2) 3. Nuclear Med (2)	Radiography will differentiate between osteoporosis-related conditions or those of other metabolic causes as characteristic signs will be evident on the images. Radiography correlates with NM to deliver increased specificity. Used with MRI it may be feasible to characterise acute and chronic porotic collapse or malignant cause for collapse rather than osteoporosis. Dual energy X-ray absorpti-ometry (DEXA) measures bone density. If hyper-trophic changes or deformity of spine makes reading DEXA difficult, consider quantitative CT as the alternative. NM can identify hypercalcae-mia seen in metastatic disease once myeloma has been excluded.

Indication	Order and investigation type (relative radiation level)	Comments
Painful osteomalacia	1. Radiography (1) 2. Nuclear Med (2) 3. MRI (0)	Closely collimated radiography may establish the cause of localised pain or support NM when equivocal. Increased activity or local complications patterns are revealed by NM; usually includes pseudofractures. MRI will identify localised bone pain causes when not revealed or equivocal using radiography.
Vertebral osteoporotic collapse	1. Radiography (1) (lateral thoracolumbar spine) 2. MRI (0) 3. DEXA (1)	Radiography is the initial test to identify osteoporotic collapsed vertebrae. MRI differentiates acute and chronic episodes and identifies malignant rather than osteoporotic causes. DEXA is not necessary in the elderly if plain radiography has established the diagnosis. DEXA should be performed to establish bone density in those with risk factors. Other abnormalities will be detected by radiography and MRI.

(*Continued*)

Indicated Imaging

Indication	Order and investigation type (relative radiation level)	Comments
Joints		
Joint disease: initial presentation	1. Radiography (diseased joint) (1) 1. Radiography (hands/ feet) (1) 2. Radiography (multiple joints) (2) 3. US (0) 4. Nuclear Med (2) 5. MRI (0)	Radiography is used to identify cause of joint problem; changes such as erosion are late features. Rheumatoid arthritis should be evaluated with feet and hand radiography. Symptomatic hands may appear normal; feet may show erosions. Radiography should be used to evaluate the symptomatic joints only. US shows acute synovitis and early erosions. Acute synovitis is evident though distribution of disease is best revealed with NM. MRI shows acute synovitis, early erosions and articular cartilage integrity.
Joint disease: follow-up	1. Radiography (1) 2. US (0) 3. MRI (0)	Radiography may be requested by specialists as a management aid. Disease progression is assessed using all 3 modalities and results employed in treatment choices. There is variation in investigation choice and much is still to be agreed with respect to best approaches.

Indication	Order and investigation type (relative radiation level)	Comments
Shoulder pain: ? impingement or rotator cuff tear	1. US (0) 2. MRI (0) 3. Radiography (1)	US will show the rotator cuff and surrounding soft tissues well and may be used for guiding injection procedures. It may be used preoperatively to establish cuff integrity, especially in cases unresponsive to initial treatment or injection. MRI complements US and is especially useful after major trauma to the shoulder. As MRI delineates abnormalities hidden by the acromion or other bone anomalies, MRI can be used to deliver a diagnosis where other modalities fail. Radiography is effective as a preoperative evaluative technique. It can be used to delineate causes for persistent shoulder pain unresponsive to conservative treatment, such as calcific tendonitis or non rotator-cuff-related problems.
Instability of shoulder	1. Radiography (1) 2. MR/MR arthrogram (0) 3. CT/CT arthrogram (2)	Instability-linked bone and joint changes are shown on radiographs. MR can show the glenoid labrum without contrast but its addition enables clear visualisation of the labrum and ligaments. The bony components of the glenoid are well revealed with CT. Addition of contrast media enables recognition of labral tears.

(Continued)

Indicated Imaging

Indication	Order and investigation type (relative radiation level)	Comments
Pain in the sacro-iliac joints	1. Radiography (1) 2. MRI (0) 3. CT (2) 4. Nuclear Med (2)	For those with seronegative arthropathy, radiography is the first-line investigative choice. Early stage sacro-iliitis is shown by MRI but without ionising radiation. CT and NM are alternative approaches that may be used.
Hip pain: no trauma	1. Radiography (1) 2. MRI (0) 3. Nuclear Med (2)	Persistent pain (focal in nature) caused by joint change, erosive arthropathy or other pathology is shown clearly on X-ray. If radiography is negative for persistent pain, MRI should be performed to evaluate further. NM may be performed but is less specific; choose MRI if available.
Possible avascular necrosis (AVN) hip pain	1. Radiography (1) 2. MRI (0) 3. Nuclear Med (2) 4. CT (2)	Radiography commonly shows normal appearance between 6/12 and 9/12 of disease onset; afterwards appearances become abnormal. MRI detects AVN early in the evolution and defines the extent clearly. NM or CT will detect AVN but with less specificity than MRI. If MRI available, choose this modality.

Indicated Imaging

Indication	Order and investigation type (relative radiation level)	Comments
Nontrauma painful knee; no locking or ↓ ROM	1. MRI (0) 2. US (0) 3. Radiography (1)	MRI is capable of delineating AVN and sepsis as causes for persistent pain without diagnosed cause. US shows causes such as tendinopathy or bursitis in the anterior knee. Soft tissues are a main cause for knee pain and these do not show well on radiographs. Osteoarthritis is a common cause for pain (shown well) and radiography is employed presurgically. If sudden onset or increasing of pain and if pain exists for over 6 weeks in children or young adults then radiographs should be obtained.
Painful knee + locking	1. MRI (0) 2. Radiography (1)	Meniscal tears and loose bodies are clearly identified on MRI and are causes of locking. Radio-opaque loose bodies will show on radiographs but these are less frequent as a cause of locking.
Pain in a prosthesis	1. Radiography (1) 2. Nuclear Med (3) 3. US (0) 4. Arthrography + biopsy/aspiration (2) 5. MRI (0)	Loosening peri-prosthetically is clearly seen on radiographs. Loosening, e.g. due to infection can be excluded with a clear NM skeletal scan. NM has limited capability in defining sterile or infective causes for loosening. US is helpful as a guide if aspiration is performed. Ultrasonic images will reveal peri-prosthetic abscesses or surface-based infective collections. Aspiration of joint fluids.
Hallux valgus	1. Radiography (1)	Radiography is used as a presurgical guide.

(Continued)

Indicated Imaging

Indication	Order and investigation type (relative radiation level)	Comments
Plantar fasciitis (heel pain)	1. Nuclear Med (2) 2. US (0) 3. MRI (0) 4. Radiography (1)	Imaging commonly dose not add to the management process. Patients should be treated clinically without relying on imaging. NM, MRI and US are able to show inflammatory changes. Calcaneal spurs are a common finding but not necessarily linked to the pain, the cause for which is rarely demonstrated by radiography.
Soft tissues		
Soft tissue masses	1. MRI (0) 2. US (0) 3. Radiography (1) 4. Biopsy + image guidance (1 or 2)	Some tissue diagnosis is achievable with MRI. Its strength is local staging. Cystic and solid masses lend themselves to US imaging. Haematomata or local recurrence of soft tissue sarcomas are also well seen. Radiography shows soft tissue calcification and/or bone masses linked with soft tissue lesions. CT may also help delineate. Deep-seated tumours are often biopsied using US guidance.
Congenital abnormalities		
Congenital disorders	1. MRI (0) 2. Radiography (1)	MRI is able to define spinal abnormalities and exclude lesions of the spinal cord/theca. Young patients may require sedation or even general anaesthetic. CT helps to visualise the bony components. Full-length spinal examination, e.g. for scoliosis, lend themselves to radiographic evaluation.

Indicated Imaging

Indication	Order and investigation type (relative radiation level)	Comments
Myelopathy		
Spinal cord disorders, e.g. tumours, infarction, inflammatory change, infection	1. MRI (0) 2. CT (2) 3. CT myelography (2) 4. Nuclear Med (2)	Spinal cord lesions should be initially investigated using MRI. It is also useful to assess cord compression and staging postoperatively. CT will add bone details if required. CT myelography should only be attempted if MRI unavailable or contraindicated in the patient. Metastatic bone disease can be screened for using NM or to identify/characterise focal lesions, e.g. osteoid osteoma.

INDICATED EXAMINATIONS FOR THE DIAGNOSIS OF CHEST AND CARDIOVASCULAR SYSTEM PRESENTATIONS

Indication	Order and investigation type (relative radiation level)
Cardiovascular system	
ST elevated myocardial infarction (STEMI) + acute chest pain	1. Radiograph – CXR (1) 2. Catheter angiography +/– intervention (3) 3. Echocardiography (0) 4. CT chest (2) 5. Nuclear Med myocardial perfusion (2) 6. MRI heart (0)
Acute chest pain, non-STEMI + unstable angina	1. Echocardiography (0) 2. Nuclear Med myocardial perfusion (2) 3. CT coronary angiography (2) 4. MRI (0) 5. Catheter coronary angiography (3)
? Aortic dissection/aortic syndrome	1. Radiograph – CXR (1) 2. CT 3. Transoesophageal echocardiography (TOE) (0) 4. MRI (0)

Comments
CXR not performed if it delays intervention – helps provide alternative diagnosis, e.g. aortic dissection or if suspicion of associated pulmonary oedema. Coronary angiography + angioplasty in centres with the service is indicated. Thrombolysis + angioplasty in myocardial rescue situations. Echo can clarify aortic dissection suspicion or confirm STEMI with bundle branch block or ? posterior MI. Can assess mechanical complications post MI. If coronary arteries normal, use CT to differentiate aortic dissection, pulmonary embolism or pericarditis. NM is used for post-thrombolysis future MI risk assessment if patient stable. Moderate stenosis risk can also be assessed. Post-revascularisation MRI may be used to assess ventricular function, degree of infarction and transmural infarct magnitude. Also used to investigate chest pain in raised troponin situations but normal coronary arteries, e.g. myocarditis, pericarditis.
Assists in evaluation of ongoing ischaemia, prognosis in left ventricular function and detection of aortic stenosis or hypertrophic cardiomyopathy. ECG-gated SPECT is used to diagnose and prognose those with intermediate risk and low or no cardiac enzymes. Can be used to further assess impact of coronary angiographic lesions. CT has a high negative predictive value for coronary artery disease (CAD) so is useful in low to intermediate risk patients. It will also detect aortic dissection, pulmonary embolism and infection or pericarditis etc. No Ca^{2+} is a good prognostic indicator for no coronary artery disease. Significance of CAD can be assessed with ECG-gated MRI using rest perfusion +/– pharmacological stress, ventricle function and delayed contrast imaging. Other pain causes can be identified when patient has low to intermediate risk but are haemodynamically stable. Indicated procedure for patients with recurrent symptoms or ischaemia despite medical intervention and are at high risk.
Used mainly to exclude other causes – not normally diagnostic. CT is the most reliable and available with non-contrast initial images able to delineate intramural haematoma. TOE works well for type A dissection+ intramural haematoma, aortic root involvement or acute aortic valve regurgitation. Local expertise and availability dictates choice between CT and TOE. Acute presentations make MRI difficult procedurally but good for sequential follow-up and aortic valve function assessment. Can be used (TOE as substitute) if iodinated contrast media prevents other modality use.

(Continued)

Indication	Order and investigation type (relative radiation level)
Cardiovascular system	
? Pulmonary embolism (PE)	*Local agreed protocols should be developed for investigation of PE suspicion with leg US providing further evidence of thromboembolism if equivocal results to that point.*
	1. Radiograph – CXR (1) 2. CT pulmonary angiogram (CTPA) (3) 3. Nuclear Med – ventilation + perfusion (2) 4. Magnetic resonance angiography (MRA) (0)
Chronic stable angina	1. Radiograph – CXR (1) 2. Echocardiography (0) 3. CT (3) 4. MRI + vasodilator or inotropic stressors (0) 5. Nuclear Med perfusion + stress (2) 6. Coronary angiography (2)
Heart valve disease	1. Echocardiography (0) 2. Radiograph – CXR (1) 3. MRI (0) 4. CT

Comments
Normal CXR does not exclude PE but should detect effusion or consolidation. CTPA is the ideal investigation in high suspicion of PE +/− pre-existing pulmonary disease. NM ventilation and perfusion may be used instead of CTPA when no pre-existing cardiopulmonary disease and CXR normal. Normal perfusion NM excludes clinically significant emboli. Consider for use if CTPA contraindicated or if NM less helpful such as in an abnormal CXR.
CXR is used to assess heart size, ventricular aneurysm, ? pulmonary congestion, pericardial Ca^{2+} and aortic aneurysm. Non cardiac chest pain causes may be revealed. Rest echo is used if a murmur ? aortic stenosis, mitral regurgitation or hypertrophic cardiomyopathy. Mural motion abnormality assessment if done within 30 minutes of pain, stress echo + dobutamine/exercise may detect ischaemia in those with intermediate CAD risk. CT coronary artery Ca^{2+} matches the exercise ECG in intermediate-risk CAD patients as significant lumen obstruction is probably linked with calcification. CTCA is useful in bypass graft obstruction evaluation. As a test it is likely to be most useful in low to medium risk CAD patients but needs a minimum 16-slice CT system. With no MRI contraindications, MRI + vasodilator stress frequently matches coronary angiography, PET and SPECT or as a replacement to stress echo when imaging is weak as the acoustic window is poor. NM will identify ischaemic areas and assess risk in those of intermediate CAD probability. At rest ECG-gated studies show left ventricle function +/− regional motion abnormalities. Gold standard examination for CAD diagnosis especially with high probability of angina, or abnormal and equivocal results from non-invasive procedures.
Current standard for detection and evaluation. If acoustic window poor or infective endocarditis try TOE. Baseline evaluation technique – shows valve Ca^{2+} cardiomegaly, pulmonary oedema/vascular congestion. Complements echocardiography if acoustic window poor and TOE not possible. If echo and catheter angiography conflict MRI may help. MRI helps in regurgitant valves and can be used in ventricular volume, function and myocardial mass. Most prosthetic valves are MR safe unless severely broken down. ECG gating with CT enables aortic valve assessment in ? aortic stenosis with Ca^{2+} related to severity in degenerative disease of the valve.

Indicated Imaging

(*Continued*)

Indication	Order and investigation type (relative radiation level)
Heart failure/myocarditis	1. Echocardiography (0) 2. Radiograph – CXR (1) 3. Nuclear Med (cardiac) 4. MRI (0) 5. CT
Congenital heart disease (CHD)	1. Echocardiography (0) 2. Radiograph – CXR (1) 3. MRI (0) 4. CT
Abdominal aortic aneurysm (AAA)	1. US (0) 2. CT (3) 3. MRI (0)
Ischaemic lower limb	1. Angiography (DSA) (3) 2. CTA (3) 3. MRA (0)
Ischaemic upper limb	1. Angiography (DSA) (3)
Deep vein thrombosis (DVT)	1. US (0) 2. Venography (2)

Comments

First-choice examination to diagnose and identify cause of failure or cardiomyopathy. Dobutamine (low-dose) stress testing will assess for cardiac hibernation if chronic ischaemic cardiomyopathy suspected.

Forms a useful control picture but normal CXR does not exclude failure. CXR used for cardiac size investigation, pulmonary congestion or associated pulmonary disease.

Multiple gating or rest SPECT with Tc99m agents are used to evaluate ejection fraction as with MRI approaches. Hibernation evaluated with Tc99m nitrates and rest redistribution + thallium-201 show hibernation. FDG-PET for metabolism + ammonia for perfusion also demonstrates cardiac hibernation.

Complements echo but better at showing ventricular volume, ejection fraction and separating ischaemic from non-ischaemic myopathy. Hibernation studies use delayed enhancement techniques or low-dose dobutamine stress tests. Test of choice for myocarditis but may reveal causes such as sarcoid or amyloidosis and iron overload/haemachromatosis.

Coronary artery CTA studies may also perform ventricular function at the same time. The technique closely matches echo (3D) MRI and ECG-gated SPECT with cardiomyopathy assessment techniques also surfacing.

Preferred technique for diagnosis and evaluation with support provided by MRI and/or CT where necessary.

Cardiac shape on CXR may imply diagnosis but mainly aids pulmonary vascular and cardiac situs identification.

Alternative approach in newborns and young children where echo is less successful; particularly helpful for complex congenital disease. MRI used in adults as postsurgical evaluation in aortic and pulmonary artery abnormalities or shunt evaluation and measurement. Nowadays most prosthetic cardiac valves are safe – older ball and cage devices or valve seat breakdown suspicions would preclude use of MRI.

CT may define complex cardiac composition if MRI not possible; will also delineate coronary artery, aortic and pulmonary vasculature though functional capability in CT for these cases is limited.

Diagnosis and sizing (diameter) of the aneurysm if the prime role of US.

CT should be used with suspected leak IF urgent surgery is not delayed.

MRI and CT display renal and iliac vessels to advantage. Good anatomical rendition is required for intravascular stenting approaches.

Due to surgical salvage requirements policy regarding proceeding with DSA should be developed with regard to possible radiological therapeutic involvement. US may be a first-line investigation.

CTA and MRA are becoming choice methods for diagnosis.

Note comment for lower limb and surgical or radiological intervention.

Most clinically significant thrombi will be detected, especially with colour flow Doppler. Other lesions may also be evident; calf thrombi detection with US has gained massive popularity.

Venography should be resorted to when US experience is limited or therapy strategy policy indicates.

(Continued)

Indication	Order and investigation type (relative radiation level)
Employment or screening medicals	1. Radiograph – CXR (1)
Preop CXR	1. Radiograph – CXR (1)
Upper respiratory tract infection (URTI)	1. Radiograph – CXR (1)
Asthma (acute) exacerbation	1. Radiograph – CXR (1)
COPD (acute) exacerbation	1. Radiograph – CXR (1)
Pneumonia	1. Radiograph – CXR (1)
Pneumonia follow-up	1. Radiograph – CXR (1)
Pleural effusion	1. Radiograph – CXR (1) 2. US (0) 3. CT (3)
Haemoptysis	1. Radiograph – CXR (1) 2. CT (3) 3. Angiography (DSA) (3)
ICU/HDU	1. Radiograph – CXR (1)
Diffuse or infiltrating lung disease	1. CT (3)

Comments
Should only be performed in the high-risk immigrant, i.e. no recent CXR = ? TB, or for occupational requirements such as deep sea divers, or for emigration requirements.
Should not be requested in <60 yrs patient unless known complications. May be increased pick-up rate in >60 yrs but if known cardiorespiratory disease detection is relatively low for other conditions.
Not indicated.
Not indicated unless life-threatening and response to treatment is inadequate. If localisation signs to region of chest, fever or increased white cell count then CXR recommended.
Should be performed if patient requires hospital referral.
Community acquired pneumonias should be followed with CXR and show resolution between 4 and 6 weeks. This may be longer in smokers, the elderly and those with chronic airway disease. For children, failure to respond to treatment or severely ill individuals indicates need for CXR. Simple pneumonia does not require routine CXR follow-up.
If clinical recovery satisfactory from community acquired pneumonia, follow-up CXR not required before hospital discharge. If persistent symptoms or physical signs at 6 weeks, or those with increased potential for neoplastic disease (>50 yrs, smoker) CXR should be arranged whether admitted to hospital or not.
Erect CXR may detect small pleural collections. US is better than CT at showing fluid loculation or internal septation after detection characterisation of pleural fluid. US may detect pleural metastases and is used to guide thoracentesis. CT aids detection and characterisation of pleural collections whilst also identify underlying pleural disease.
A CXR is mandatory in these cases. If normal CXR with significant haemoptysis further examination (CT if imaging) should be performed. CT (+/− CTA) and bronchoscopy are used together. CT will define malignant or nonmalignant disease not seen with CXR or bronchoscopy. CT will NOT detect submucosal problems. Selective bronchial catheter angiography +/− embolisation may be a life-saving intervention in massive haemoptysis.
CXRs are helpful with a change in symptoms or after devices are inserted, exchanged or removed. Daily CXR is now in question and CT may be employed to solve problems in critically ill patients.
High resolution CT (HRCT) has been shown to be equivalent to histology in disease identification and providing prognostic information about reversibility of disease.

Indicated Imaging

INDICATED EXAMINATIONS FOR THE DIAGNOSIS OF COMMON GASTROINTESTINAL PRESENTATIONS

Indication	Order and investigation type (relative radiation level)
Upper gastrointestinal tract	
Upper oesophagus dysphagia	1. Barium swallow (2) 2. Video fluoroscopy (2)
Lower oesophagus dysphagia	1. Barium swallow (2) 2. Nuclear Med (2)
Oesophageal reflux, hiatus hernia or chest pain	1. Barium swallow and meal (2)
? Oesophageal perforation	1. Chest X-ray (1) 2. Contrast medium swallow (2) 3. CT (3)
Acute GI bleeding, haematemesis or melaena	1. Endoscopy (0) 2. US (0) 3. CT (3) 4. CT angiography (2) 5. Nuclear Med (3) (red cell labelled) 6. Angiography (3) 7. Radiograph (1) 8. Barium studies (2)

Indicated Imaging

Comments
Even with normal endoscopy there may be motility problems. Barium studies should be performed prone, supine and erect. Endoscopically occult strictures are revealed by barium + bolus studies. Recording of the swallowing mechanism is required + speech therapist and ENT surgeon is ideal.
In the >40 years patient with dysphagia that began recently and has progressed, endoscopy is the investigation of choice. High dysphagia is shown as indicated above. Barium will displays pouches and webs. A radionuclide transit study of the oesophagus my replace the barium motility study.
Investigation should occur following non-response to treatment and/or lifestyle changes due to reflux. Endoscopy shows the early changes of oesophagitis and demonstrates metaplasia that may be biopsied. pH monitoring best defines reflux and barium examinations are most useful prior to surgery to assess motility. They do not forecast the potential for post-surgical dysphagia.
Radiography of the chest will show abnormality in 80% of cases. A pneumomediastinum will be visible in only 60%. Use diluted nonionic iodinated contrast media as this is safest; if no leak visible, CT should be performed. CT will detect oesophageal perforation and show mediastinal or pleural complications.
Identification and haemostatic treatment of upper GIT bleeding is possible with endoscopy. Chronic liver disease may be a cause of haematemesis; US will delineate this problem well. CT and CTA may be used to diagnose acute GIT bleeding. Nuclear medicine should be performed after endoscopy. Red cell labelling may detect flow rates as low as 0.1 mL/min, which is more sensitive than angiographic imaging. If bleeding cannot be stopped angiography may be used to identify the source or guide surgery; alternatively embolisation via catheter is a possible management approach. Plain radiography adds nothing to patient management. If barium studies are performed (not appropriate) angiographic procedures cannot be employed afterwards.

(*Continued*)

Indicated Imaging

Indication	Order and investigation type (relative radiation level)
Dyspepsia	1. Barium studies (2) 2. US (0)
Chronic or recurrent GIT bleeding	1. Barium meal/enema (2/2) 2. Small bowel enteroclysis (2) 3. Nuclear Med (2) (red cell label/Meckels study) 4. CT (3) 5. Angiography (3)
Acute abdominal pain ? Perforation ? Obstruction	1. Radiograph (1) 2. Abdomen + erect chest (1) 3. US (0) 4. CT (3)
Acute small bowel obstruction	1. Contrast radiography (2) 2. CT (3) 3. Radiography (1) 4. US (0)
Small bowel disease, e.g. Crohn's	1. Small bowel meal (2) 2. Small bowel enema (2) 3. Endoscopy/video capsule (0) 4. US (0) 5. CT (3) 6. MRI (0) 7. Nuclear Med (white cell) (3)

Comments

Endoscopy is the first-choice investigation following unsuccessful trial therapies. A diagnosis of gallstones should be ruled out if endoscopy and barium studies are normal. In the >55 years patient, persistent recently starting dyspepsia should result in an endoscopy request. Endoscopy should be performed on any age person with dyspepsia and/or: continued unintended weight loss, progressive dysphagia, persistent vomiting, chronic GIT bleeding, iron-deficiency anaemia. Barium meal should be employed if patient refuses endoscopy and may diagnose functional dyspepsia when −ve endoscopy.

US will diagnose gallstone disease to support a −ve endoscopy or barium meal to investigate dyspepsia.

Endoscopy should be supplemented with barium meal or enema if upper and lower GIT is −ve using direct visual techniques. Small lesions may be best detected with small bowel enteroclysis. Video capsule technology may be employed for indistinct bleeding patterns that may recur after −ve endoscopy.

Labelled red cells or Meckels studies may be performed by NM when detection and localisation of chronic/recurrent bleeding proves difficult.

Intravenous contrast-enhanced CT can demonstrate lesions that are actively bleeding, e.g. tumours. CT angiography may be used to show angiodysplasias.

Angiography is sensitive for angiodysplasias and neovascularisation of tumours.

CT is beginning to take over as the initial examination BUT supine AXR shows diagnosis + anatomical position. Erect AXR should only be performed if clinical obstruction but nil on supine AXR. Free gas is best revealed on erect CXR with lateral decubitus as alternative when CXR must be supine.

US is grossly affected by body habitus and operator but will show free fluid post-perforation, identifies bowel disease and will show appendicitis.

Sealed perforation or anatomical delineation of obstruction site are suited to CT exploration. This is not appropriate in children however.

Delayed plain images up to 6 hrs post oral contrast will predict resolution without operative investigation.

CT will confirm the diagnosis of small bowel obstruction seen on plain radiography. CT enteroclysis gives site sensitivity and specificity when AXR uncertain or low-grade obstruction is clinically suspected.

US may be employed to show functional or obstructive ileus by viewing peristalsis – CT is more consistent in its diagnosis.

CT (adults) and US (paediatrics/young females) are superseding barium studies. Video capsule approach must only be used if strictures have been ruled out.

CT, US and MRI are gradually being used more in disease assessment with particular gains in extralumen lesions.

Labelled white cell studies complements barium examinations to show extent of disease through white cell generated radioactivity.

Indicated Imaging

(Continued)

Indication	Order and investigation type (relative radiation level)
Lower gastrointestinal tract	
Acute colonic obstruction	1. Radiograph – abdomen (1) 2. Contrast enema (3) 3. CT (3)

Acute pain
  intensification + inflammatory
  bowel disease
	1. Radiograph – abdomen (1)
	2. Contrast enema (3)
	3. CT (3)
	4. Nuclear Med (white cells) (3)
	5. MRI (0)

Long-term follow-up of inflammatory bowel disease	1. Barium enema (3) 2. CT colonography (3)
Acute abdomen pain ? surgery	1. Radiography – abdomen + erect chest (1) 2. US (0) 3. CT (3)
Conspicuous masses	1. Radiograph – abdomen (1) 2. US (0) 3. CT (3)
Constipation	1. Radiograph – abdomen (1) 2. Transit studies (2) 3. Proctography (2) 4. MRI (0)

Unknown pyrexia + abdominal
  sepsis
	1. US (0)
	2. CT (3)
	3. Nuclear Med (white cells,
	  gallium or PET) (3)

Comments
Clinical suspicion and level of obstruction is supported by AXR appearances. Significant obstructing lesions may be missed despite potential for these studies to confirm presence and level of obstruction. Pseudo-obstruction may be indicated in difficult-to-interpret imaging. In possible stenting cases enemas of this nature are suggested to support procedure. CT may be used as an adjunct to enemas to confirm presence, level and cause for colonic obstruction.
The plain AXR is used to monitor toxic dilatation of the bowel. Use of the non-prepared enema will confirm disease magnitude, but is contraindicated with toxic megacolon. CT helps delineate complications such as abscesses or bowel perforation. Labelled white cell studies demonstrate extent of disease. MRI supports decision-making in surgical management for anorectal infective cases.
Barium enema often fails to fully evaluate following complex surgery and visualisation of fistulae. Dysplasia, stricture and cancer are best revealed with colonoscopy which is also the preferred method of evaluation. CT colonography may replace colonoscopy if it is not feasible as an investigative approach.
Supine AXR gas patterns will reveal significant information with erect AXR performed when supine equivocal. Erect CXR will identify free gas of perforation. Biliary or gynaecological origin pain is best revealed with US with CT providing the widest range of information using a single procedure.
Plain abdominal radiography rarely aids diagnosis. US will be very helpful in detecting and characterising without the use of ionising radiation. CT will support uncertain US results; it will also demonstrate disease extent as a staging procedure before treatment is initiated.
Extent of faecal impaction is clearly revealed on radiographs. Most useful in geriatric and psychiatric presentations. Ingested radio-opaque pellets are followed using time sequence abdominal radiographs. Constipation may be a follow-on disorder of evacuation. This fluoroscopic procedure can be used to characterise the problem. Pelvic floor weaknesses are revealed with dynamic MRI. Urinary bladder herniations (cystocoeles) may also be demonstrated.
With localising signs US should be used first to gain definitive diagnoses. It is most helpful in the pelvis and subdiaphragmatic or subhepatic areas. Infection or neoplasia can be identified or rejected as causes. CT has more value during biopsy and collection drainage, especially after recent surgery where US is difficult to achieve. When no localising characteristics NM with white cell labelling will show chronic postoperative infections. Gallium can be used to reveal tumours and infections.

Indicated Imaging

(*Continued*)

Indication	Order and investigation type (relative radiation level)
Hepato/pancreato/biliary system	
Liver secondaries	1. US (0) 2. CT (3) 3. MRI (0) 4. PET-CT (4)
Solitary liver lesion characterisation	1. CT (3) 2. MRI (0) 3. US + contrast (0)
Cirrhotic complications	1. US (0) 2. CT (3) 3. MRI (0)
Jaundice	1. US (0) 2. ERCP (2) 3. CT (3) 4. MRI (+MRCP) (0) 5. US (endoscopic) 6. Percutaneous transhepatic cholangiogram (PTC)

Indicated Imaging

Comments

US will detect liver secondaries but is not reliable in their exclusion (CT or MRI provides more accurate staging). US + contrast will elevate detection to levels consistent with CT and MRI.
CT is more sensitive at detecting small lesions invisible to US. In liver resection candidates, CT is modality of choice to stage for metastatic disease.
MRI + liver-specific contrast will spot and characterise smaller lesions than CT. Again, preoperative staging prior to liver resection in patients able to tolerate MRI also makes this a modality of choice.
Specialised procedure that is beginning to prove useful in guiding liver resections.

Availability and expertise govern the use of MRI or CT in single lesion characterisation.
US + contrast is accurate in excluding malignancy and delineating focal lesions.

US is sensitive for ascites and revealing varices in portal hypertension. US is improved as a technique if + contrast so will detect and affirm hepatoma presence.
If staging for hepatoma and alpha feto-protein is raised, with uncertain US, the 3-phase CT should be used.
MRI will detect hepatoma more readily than CT in the cirrhotic liver.

(Non)obstructive jaundice is detected and differentiated with US. Further imaging depends on the presence of biliary calculi in the gallbladder or ducts and level of obstruction and clinical presentation. Duct dilation may be subtle at first and not always detected with US.
US + duct calculi = ERCP to confirm and provide intervention. Iatrogenic pancreatitis may follow ERCP intervention.
If US shows obstruction is below the hilum, CT is used to provide pancreatic cancer staging for resection. If obstruction is hilar, CT is used to plan surgery or palliative treatment.
MRCP should be attempted before ERCP if US shows no duct calculi. If hilar-level obstruction, MRCP shows pattern and extent of ductal involvement for planning of intervention. If malignant, MRI aids definition of surgical planning or defines palliative approach or otherwise.
Endoscopically performed US is highly accurate at detecting small ductal calculi as well as tumours in and around the ampulla of Vater. Pancreatic biopsy minus tumour seeding is possible with this method.
Where ERCP is not possible, direct percutaneous transhepatic catheterisation (under imaging control) will provide biliary system information. It may also be performed alongside percutaneous interventions/therapies.

Indicated Imaging

(*Continued*)

Indication	Order and investigation type (relative radiation level)
Gallbladder disease or post cholecystectomy pain	1. US (0) 2. CT (3) 3. ERCP (2) 4. MRCP (0) 5. US (endoscopic) (0) 6. Nuclear Med (2) 7. Radiograph – abdomen (1)
Post-surgery biliary leak	1. US (0) 2. MRCP (0) 3. ERCP (2) 4. Nuclear Med (2)
Acute pancreatitis	1. Radiograph – abdomen and chest (1) 2. CT (3) 3. US (0)
Chronic pancreatitis	1. Radiograph – abdomen (1) 2. US (0) 3. CT (3) 4. ERCP (2) 5. MRCP (0)

Indicated Imaging

Comments

Investigation of choice for biliary pain, gallstones or ? acute cholecystitis but US does not consistently exclude all common bile duct calculi.
Gallbladder tumours, gallbladder wall lesions are best revealed by CT. CT also does not reveal all ductal calculi but CT cholangiography is an acceptable alternative in patients unable to tolerate MRCP.
MRCP should be used to diagnose over ERCP. If previous imaging suggests biliary system disease that can be therapeutically managed with ERCP, then ERCP should be performed without MRCP.
Endoscopic US will detect very small ductal calculi and should be used if other imaging is negative but clinical suspicion is high.
NM is a useful adjunct procedure when US does not reveal acute cholcystitis, gallbladder dysfunction or problems with the sphincter of Oddi.
Abdominal radiography is limited in use, especially as 10% or fewer calculi are visible on plain radiographs.

US will show the position and size of collections associated with leaks and should be the first line of investigation.
Bile duct anatomy +/– evidence of leakage will be revealed on MRCP.
ERCP should only be pursued in these cases if it has therapeutic potential.
An HIDA study will show increased radioactivity at the site of the leaking anastomosis.

AXR and CXR are used to exclude other causes (perforation, obstruction) for the acute abdominal presentation that is causing the pain.
CT + contrast will assess degree of necrosis to enable prognostic evaluation. Follow-up CT will detect and stage any complications and is more sensitive and specific in these cases than US.
Gallstone pancreatitis will be revealed if US occurs early in the disease process. MRCP and/or ERCP, depending on the therapeutic potential, may also be considered early in the development of disease. Pancreatic US may be normal early in the disease process.

The AXR is of limited value as fewer than 10% of biliary duct calculi will be visible.
Thinner patients enhance the capability of US in pancreatic investigations.
CT will detect pancreatic calcifications but is less sensitive in early pancreatic tissue changes. US, CT and MR are poor differentiators of chronic inflammatory and malignant neoplastic masses.
ERCP shows duct morphology. ERCP should follow CT or MRCP where these modalities are equivocal or if ERCP therapeutic intervention is planned for the patient.
MRCP shows moderate to severe changes of the pancreatic duct to link with the exocrine function of the gland; however, it is weaker at revealing side ducts and mild pancreatic changes.

Indicated Imaging

INDICATED EXAMINATIONS FOR THE GENITOURINARY SYSTEM AND ADRENAL GLANDS

Indication	Order and investigation type (relative radiation level)
Urinary tract	
Renal failure	1. US (0) 2. Radiograph – AXR (1) 3. Nuclear Med (MAG3 or DMSA) (3) 4. MRI (0) 5. CT (3) 6. Contrast radiography – IVU (2)
Kidney transplant dysfunction	1. US + Doppler (0) 2. Nuclear Med (2) 3. MRI + MRA (0)
Renal and ureteric colic	1. CT (3) 2. Contrast radiography – IVU (2) 3. US + AXR (1) 4. MR urography (0)
Renal stones – no colic	1. AXR/CT (1/2) 2. US (0)
Renal mass	1. US (0) 2. Contrast radiography – IVU (2) 3. CT (3) 4. MRI (0)

Comments

US is the primary modality to use. It reveals dilation of the collecting system for obstructive reasoning of failure and is a biopsy guide when histology is required. Calculi may be shown using this method if not seen using US.
NM again shows level of functional drainage secondary to pelviureteric junction obstruction or relative kidney function if failure suspected.
An alternative to contrast CT though MRI media are contraindicated in renal failure.
CT supports equivocal US (esp if obstruction cause not seen ultrasonically). Poor renal function negates use of contrast media.
The IVU should not be performed.

US can assess for hydronephrosis, other collections and kidney perfusion. Colour Doppler will show transplant artery stenosis but Doppler cannot separate acute rejection from acute tubular necrosis – support with biopsy.
NM will aid diagnosis of obstruction when dilatation seen with US. Acute rejection can be differentiated from acute tubular necrosis with NM.
MRA will differentiate transplant artery stenosis where US is equivocal, but note MRI contrast is contraindicated in renal failure.

Use of a low-dose CT technique ensures multislice CT gains points in accuracy and reduced radiation use – use first.
Perform in colic situations where CT is not practicable.
US is less accurate than CT or IVU but if used in combination with AXR may be used when CT and IVU contraindicated.
Can be useful during pregnancy to confirm cause of colic with associated hydronephrosis.

The AXR or non-contrast media CT gives a good baseline evaluation of those suspected of renal calculi. AXR will detect most stones containing Ca^{2+} but non-enhanced CT is more sensitive. Follow-up examinations should repeat initial investigative method.
Though less sensitive than CT, US (and CT) can detect urate calculi.

US will see masses >2 cm and define as solid or cystic – may help characterise indeterminate masses seen on CT.
Less sensitive than US and unable to characterise masses accurately.
Masses of 1–1.5 cm are detectable with generally accurate characterisation.
MRI + contrast matches contrast-enhanced CT for detection sensitivity and characterisation. Poor renal function and hence contraindication for contrast CT or inadequate characterisation by CT or US are indicators for using MRI.

Indicated Imaging

(*Continued*)

Indication	Order and investigation type (relative radiation level)
Diagnosis of causes of renal tract obstruction	1. US (0) 2. CT (3) 3. MRI (0) 4. Contrast radiography – IVU (2) 5. Nuclear Med (2)
Infection of adult urinary tract	1. US + AXR (0 + 1) 2. CT 3. Contrast radiography – IVU (2)
Urinary retention	1. US (0) 2. Contrast radiography – IVU (2)
Prostatism	1. US (0) 2. Contrast radiography – IVU (2)
Renovascular	
Hypertension + non medical response or young adult	1. MRA (0) 2. US (0) 3. CTA (3) 4. Nuclear Med (pre & post captopril) (3) 5. DSA angiography (3) 6. Contrast radiography – IVU (2)

Indicated Imaging

Comments
US will reveal collecting system dilatation and show (with Doppler) intrarenal blood flow, the bladder and any ureteric jets. Non-contrast CT is best from ureteric colic but contrast-enhanced CT in excretory phase will show intrinsic and extrinsic urinary tract obstructive causes. MR urography is good for pregnant, paediatric patients or those with contrast allergy issues. Where the collecting system is dilated, MR can show the level and diagnosis of the cause of the problem. The IVU is used to demonstrate anatomy preoperatively should CT be unavailable. A Tc-99m-MAG3 + frusemide technique is used to show response to the diuretic that is independent of renal function. Combined with parenchymal transit time assessment, the evaluation of obstructive nephropathy is possible.
Usually most adults do not require imaging for this presentation BUT if an infection does not clear rapidly with antibiotics, immunocompromised or diabetic patients, after the proven UTI has settled in men or after 1 UTI recurrence in women then imaging would be warranted. CT can detect small calculi, renal sepsis and pyelonephritic changes not seen by US. Consider as an adjunct to US + AXR. Can be used in the non-acute phase if suspicion of other renal disease, e.g. reflux nephropathy, papillary necrosis.
Kidney imaging is advised for renal tract dilatation post-catheterisation to relieve bladder distension. Should not be performed for this presentation.
Bladder US is indicated to look at residual post-micturition residue volume and to look at flow rate. If residue is present, haematuria, raised creatinine values or suspected infection then US of kidneys is advised. Should not be performed for this presentation.
MRA is the best noninvasive visualisation method in those able to undergo MRI. Specialised examination. US with Doppler is sensitive and specific for the renal artery but is highly operator-dependent for main renal artery evaluation. CTA is as good as MRI, however relies upon iodinated contrast and high irradiation levels – only use if MRA not possible and no renal impairment. Captopril renography will pick up functionally significant renal artery stenosis. It may be used to assess kidney revascularisation in treated renal hypertension. DSA will show stenotic lesions that are being considered for surgery or angioplasty. Pressure measurement across the stenosis will aid diagnosis of functionally significant lesions. IVU is not indicated to evaluate for renal hypertension where no other renal disease is evident.

(*Continued*)

Indicated Imaging

Indication	Order and investigation type (relative radiation level)
Reproductive	
Torsion of the testis	1. US (0)
Male infertility	1. US – scrotal + transrectal (0) 2. MRI (0)
Adrenal glands	
Adrenal medullary tumour evaluation	1. US (0) 2. CT/MRI (3/0) 3. Nuclear Med (3) 3. PET CT (3)
Cushing's disease – adrenal cortical lesions	1. CT/MRI/Nuclear Med (3/0/2) (iodo cholesterol) 2. Venous sampling (3)
Primary hyperaldosteronism (Conn's syndrome) due to lesions of the adrenal cortex	1. CT/MRI (3/0)

Comments
Imaging should not delay intervention esp. if a clinical diagnosis has been made. US should be used where clinical diagnosis is equivocal and even though Colour Doppler US is sensitive for suspected torsion false negative results have been reported. Intermittent torsion continues to pose diagnostic problems.
US of the scrotum measures testicular volume, exclude pathology, define testicular texture and look for varicocoeles. Transrectal imaging will establish whether obstruction of the seminal vesicles, ejaculatory ducts or vas deferens is the cause for infertility. MRI is used to clarify any transrectal US results.
US may be more helpful for children (radiation protection for CT or unable to tolerate MRI) and may detect and incidental tumour. CT/MRI gives the best anatomical rendition of tumours and defines benign from malignant. Without biochemical changes imaging is not indicated. Functioning tumours can be located with NM, especially in ectopic or metastatic presentations. Consider PET CT in equivocal initial imaging.
Seek advice about most appropriate imaging avenue. In Cushing's syndrome CT/MRI may detect an adrenal cause BUT nodular hyperplasia is frequently the cause in ACTH-dependent and independent Cushing's. In these cases CT may define an adenoma from nodular hyperplasia but NM +/– adrenal venous sampling may be necessary to confirm.
CT and MRI are able to differentiate between adrenal adenoma and bilateral hyperplasia. Seek advice about the best examination.

Indicated Imaging

INDICATED EXAMINATIONS FOR THE DIAGNOSIS, STAGING AND FOLLOW-UP OF CANCER FOR THE MOST COMMON CANCER PRESENTATIONS (EXCLUDES SKIN CANCERS)

Area	Diagnosis	
	Investigation type	Relative radiation level
Lung	CXR	1
	CT	3
	Not all cancers will be visible on CXR despite positive sputum tests. CT has greater diagnostic sensitivity for earlier detection but its use as a screening tool is unconfirmed.	
Prostate	US	0
	Transrectal US is most common with guided biopsy.	

Staging		Follow-up	
Investigation type	**Relative radiation level**	**Investigation type**	**Relative radiation level**
CT	3		
PET-CT	4		
MRI	0		
US	0		
CT + histology = 80% accuracy in mediastinal lymph node enlargement. Consider PET-CT for further nodal detection, esp. non-small-cell lung cancer and presurgical resection/radical oncology intervention. MRI has greater value in pancoast tumours (no real difference to CT otherwise) and may help differentiate atelectasis from tumour. MRI has vascular uses for iodine-reactive patients. US helpful for FNA of neck nodes to confirm spread at early phase of diagnosis.			
MRI	0		
Nuclear Med	2		
Pelvic phased array endorectal coils in MRI provides most sensitive and specific assessment prior to radical intervention. Extension of MRI into the abdomen for pelvic node disease – transrectal US may also be of value. Nuclear Med bone scan for metastases for patients with ↑ PSA and Gleason scores. 20+ PSA and 8+ Gleason are indicators for disseminated bone disease.			

(*Continued*)

Indicated Imaging

Area	Diagnosis	
	Investigation type	**Relative radiation level**
Breast	Mammo	1
	US	0
	MRI	0
	Nuclear Med	3
	After referral to breast clinic mammo and US are part of the assessment of clinical, imaging and pathology. Mammo = good for +35yrs ♀ with US for <35yrs. MRI could augment staging when assessment not clear i.e. imaging and pathology disagree – same requirement applies for scintimammography. Breast augmentation is best evaluated in clinical suspicion in women with implants.	
Colorectal	Barium enema	3
	CT colonography	3
	Colonoscopy	0
	CT	3
	Barium enema and colonoscopy are favoured approaches depending on availability with CT colonography particularly helpful for elderly or infirm. CT colonography may be used in failed colonoscopy of insufficient bowel preparation. CT of pelvis and abdomen is useful esp. in older or infirm patients with staging performed simultaneously.	

Indicated Imaging

Staging		Follow-up	
Investigation type	Relative radiation level	Investigation type	Relative radiation level
Mammo	1	Mammo	1
CXR	1	US	0
US	0	MRI	0
Nuclear Med	3	Nuclear Med	3
CT	3	With breast conservation follow up best served by mammo, US and MRI. If possible local or regional recurrence re-do initial assessment +/– scintimammography to confirm.	
MRI	0		
Mammo + US is used for local staging with problematic lesions reserved for MRI. Distant spread is supported by Nuclear Med bone scans, CXR + liver US +/– CT of chest and abdomen as decided by breast care team.			
CXR	1	US	0
US	0	CT	3
CT	3	MRI	0
MRI	0	PET-CT	4
PET-CT	4	US and CT may be used in asymptomatic patients for continuing observation. MRI is advantageous for detecting local recurrence with PET-CT being sensitive to local and peritoneal tumour return and tumours of the colon and rectum. PET-CT is particularly helpful when imaging is normal but rising tumour markers are evident clinically.	
CXR is used in secondary pulmonary disease in palliative cases esp if CT unavailable. CT is routine for treatment decisions with US helpful in anal and rectal early stages. Liver spread may use US but CT, MRI and Pet-CT are more sensitive in hepatic secondaries. MRI is best for local spread + contrast for hepatic secondary resection with PET-CT being favoured for resectable pulmonary and hepatic metastases.			

(Continued)

Indicated Imaging

Area	Diagnosis	
	Investigation type	**Relative radiation level**
Bladder	US	0
	IVU	2
	Imaging of this nature is relatively insufficient when contrasted with cystoscopy which would be the method of choice. Lesions of under 5 mm are difficult to confirm using the above imaging methods.	
Lymphoma	CT	3
	US	0
	Excision biopsy of lymph nodes are the gold standard, however where impossible CT and US will act as guides for needle biopsy of the node.	

Staging		Follow-up	
Investigation type	**Relative radiation level**	**Investigation type**	**Relative radiation level**
CT	3		
IVU	2		
CXR	1		
MRI	0		
PET-CT	4		
CT can identify spread outside the bladder to the pelvis and is helpful to survey lymph nodes and distal secondaries in the thorax and abdomen. An IVU may diagnose multiple urothelial tumours and CXR ascertains pulmonary secondaries. MRI has high sensitivity and specificity when assessing the bladder, local spread into neighbouring organs but less helpful for distant metastatic spread. Complex problems may be addressed with PET-CT.			
CT	3	CXR	1
US	0	CT	3
MRI	0	PET-CT	4
PET-CT	4	MRI	0
CT of chest, abdomen and pelvis are routine following diagnosis with head and neck possible adjuncts. US is used for specific organs particularly neck, thyroid, testis and soft tissue masses. MRI aids CNS and bone marrow staging. PET-CT may form part of initial staging with follow-up is planned.		Response by large thoracic disease to treatment may be assessed with CXR with longer-term follow-up after treatment ends. Response to treatment is also assessed by evaluating nodal size on CT where residual mass may be visible – patients in complete remission should be investigated with CT on clinical presentation basis if relapse suspected. PET-CT is helpful during treatment to predict outcome by response measurement and to assess remaining masses. MRI is valuable for CNS disease.	

Indicated Imaging

(*Continued*)

Area	Diagnosis	
	Investigation type	**Relative radiation level**
Kidney	CXR	1
	US	0
	CT	3
	MRI	0
	IVU	2
	CXRs are most useful in pulmonary secondary spread with US being most useful for lesions >2 cm as it characterises cystic or solid status and clarifies indeterminate CT findings. CT is most sensitive for lesions 1–1.5 cm in size and usually is able to characterise abnormalities. MRI is equivalent to CT in its abilities to characterise and may clarify indeterminate CT and US findings. MRI is the best alternative where iodine-based contrast agents cannot be used. The IVU is able to detect transitional cell Ca in the calyces, pelvis and ureters.	
Endometrial (Uterine body)	US	0
	MRI	0
	MRI is more helpful in identifying lesions as benign or malignant.	
Pancreas	US	0
	CT	3
	MRI	0
	MRCP	0
	ERCP	2
	In slim patient US is of value but in larger patients the pancreas is better visualised with CT. Endoscopic US might be employed for fluid aspiration. MRI is used as a clarification tool with MRCP being used in jaundice investigations where Ca pancreas is suspected. ERCP's interventional potential is best exploited following cross-sectional imaging as this will dictate likely management possibilities.	

Staging		Follow-up	
Investigation type	**Relative radiation level**	**Investigation type**	**Relative radiation level**
CT	3	Recurrence	
MRI	0	CXR	1
PET-CT	4	CT	3
Multidetector CT is the staging imaging method of choice if iodine-based contrast agents can be tolerated. Secondaries of the chest or other distal spread can be detected with this modality with MRI being reserved for the more difficult cases, e.g. vascular definition is unclear on CT. PET-CT may be an appropriate adjunct where CT or MRI are unable to clearly delineate metastases.		The regular use of CXR is most useful for T1 or T2 stage tumours at low risk of recurrence for 5 years post-surgery. Those at risk of relapse or those with symptoms suggestive of local recurrence should have routine follow-up with abdominal CT.	
MRI	0		
CT	3		
MRI gives the best evaluation of local and pelvic node staging whereas CT may be helpful for lymph node evaluation generally.			
US	0		
CT	3		
MRI	0		
PET-CT	4		
Endoscopic US	0		
Hepatic metastases may have been detected with initial US, though for radical surgery CT provides information on vascular invasion. MRI + MRCP is a useful adjunct and PET-CT is helpful for equivocal cases where secondary spread is being considered. When resection is considered impossible with other modalities, endoscopic US can be employed to guide biopsy.			

(*Continued*)

Area	Diagnosis	
	Investigation type	**Relative radiation level**
Thyroid	US	0
	Nuclear Med	2
	US is used to guide or as a combination with FNA technique. CT is best employed to demonstrate residual or recurrent differentiated cancers of the thyroid after surgical removal of the gland.	
Oesophagus	Ba swallow	2
	Endoscopy would be the gold standard investigation. Ba swallow has a role in dysphagia high in the oesophagus.	

Staging		Follow-up	
Investigation type	**Relative radiation level**	**Investigation type**	**Relative radiation level**
MRI	0		
CT	3		
US	0		
Nuclear Med	4		
MRI, CT and US combine to assess large primary lesions, detect distant secondaries or evaluate medullary thyroid Ca where multiple endocrine syndromes are evident. Nuclear med is used to detect residual or recurrent disease following thyroidectomy.			
CT	3		
Endoscopic US	0		
PET-CT	4		
CT is helpful to identify locally advanced or secondary deposits as patients usually attend with advanced disease which may preclude surgery. CT has a role in planning therapy. Endoscopic US is good to stage a resectable primary tumour with just local/regional nodes. PET-CT is useful for distal metastases detection or residual/recurrent lesion after surgery. Accurate staging is important in treatment decisions.			

Indicated Imaging

Chapter 14

Eponymous Injuries and Classification Systems

Eponyms (and in some cases classification systems) are often confused, and it is argued by some radiologists that they should not be used. However, there are several eponyms that remain in use and these are defined here with a diagram to support. Major classification systems are also listed as these too are in use and may be confused if not fully appreciated.

AVIATOR'S ATRAGALUS

A range of talar fractures first named for World War I plane crash injuries where the rudder bar was driven into the foot.

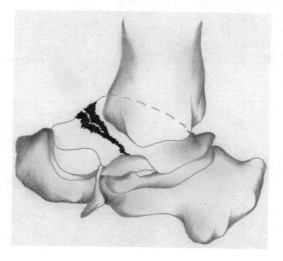

Index of Medical Imaging, First Edition. Jonathan McConnell.
© 2011 Blackwell Publishing Ltd. Published 2011 by Blackwell Publishing Ltd.

BARTON'S FRACTURE

A displaced articular lip fracture of the distal radius in either dorsal or volar orientations +/− carpal subluxation.

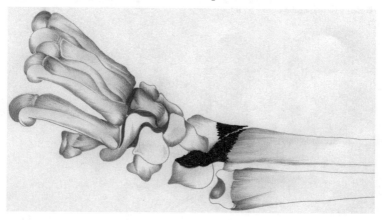

BENNETT'S FRACTURE

An oblique intra-articular first metacarpal base fracture that separates a small triangular fragment from the proximally displaced metacarpal shaft.

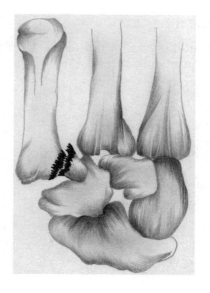

BOSWORTH'S FRACTURE

A fracture of the distal fibula resulting in displacement and fixation of the proximal fracture fragment to lie behind the postero-lateral tibial ridge.

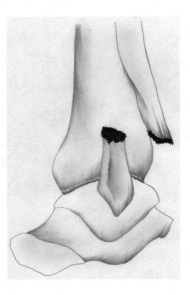

BOXER'S FRACTURE

Fracture of the neck of the fifth metacarpal with volar displacement of the metacarpal head.

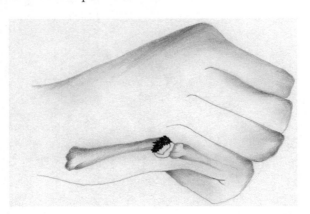

Injuries and Classification Systems

BURST FRACTURE

Vertebral body fracture due to axial loading and outward fragment displacement, often into the spinal canal of the cervical, thoracic and lumbar vertebrae.

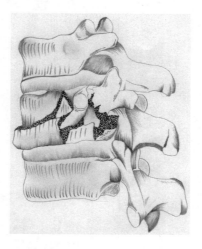

CHANCE FRACTURE

A fracture of the thoracolumbar vertebrae following distraction, to generate a horizontally disrupted spinous process, neural arch and vertebral body.

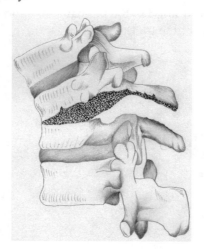

CHAUFFEUR'S FRACTURE (HUTCHINSON'S FRACTURE)

An oblique intra-articular fracture of the radial styloid, initially attributed to a starting handle being forcibly reversed during a backfire.

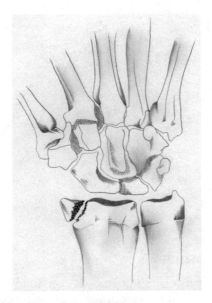

CHOPART'S FRACTURE DISLOCATION

Fracture +/− dislocation of the talonavicular and calcaneocuboid joints (Chopart) of the foot.

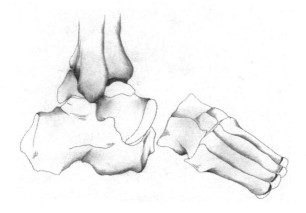

Injuries and Classification Systems

CLAY/COAL SHOVELLER'S FRACTURE

A lower cervical or upper thoracic spinous process fracture, initially attributed to workers trying to throw a shovelful of clay upwards with the clay adhering to the shovel. A resultant flexion force opposite to the neck musculature generates a fracture.

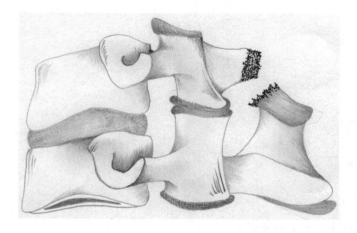

COLLES FRACTURE

A generalised description of distal radial fracture (+/− ulnar styloid fracture) with dorsal displacement of the distal fracture fragment. The Frykman classification fully describes.

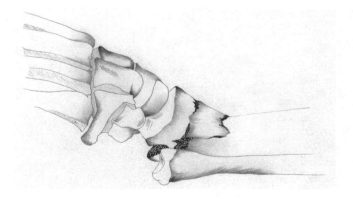

COTTON'S FRACTURE

A trimalleolar fracture of both malleoli plus a posterior tibial lip injury.

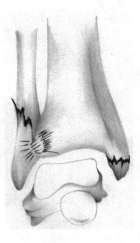

DUPUYTREN'S FRACTURE

Fracture of the distal fibula and rupture of the distal tibiofibular ligament to allow lateral displacement of the talus.

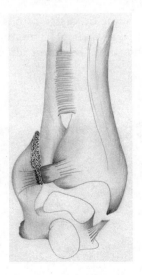

DUVERNEY'S FRACTURE

Iliac wing fracture minus pelvic ring disruption.

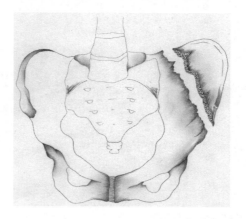

GALEAZZI'S FRACTURE

A distal third radial fracture with distal radioulnar joint subluxation.

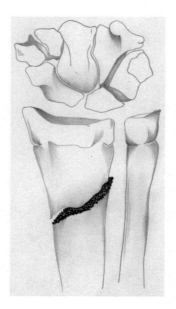

GREENSTICK FRACTURE

An incomplete fracture in a child's bone where the cortex and periosteum remain intact on the compression side of the injury.

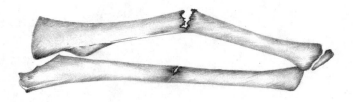

HAHN-STEINTHAL FRACTURE

A fracture that results in shearing off of a large portion of the capitellum +/− trochlear involvement.

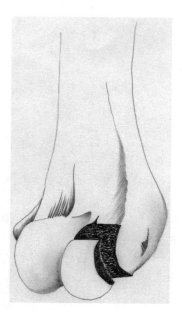

Injuries and Classification Systems

HANGMAN'S FRACTURE

Fracture through the neural arch of the second cervical vertebra (may also be termed traumatic spondylolisthesis of C2 and could have C3 component involvement due to force direction).

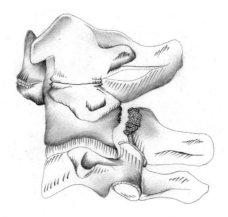

HILL-SACH'S FRACTURE (LESION)

A compression fracture of the posterolateral portion of the humeral head. Follows anterior glenohumeral dislocation with humeral head impaction against the glenoid rim.

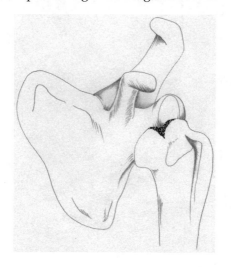

JEFFERSON'S FRACTURE

A comminuted compression fracture of the C1 ring (e.g. shallow water diving injury) with injuries usually seen anterior and posterior to the lateral facet joints.

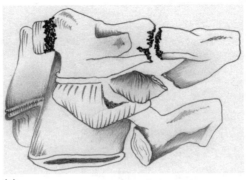

(a)

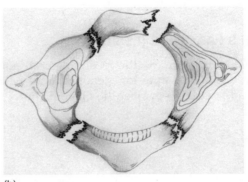

(b)

LISFRANC FRACTURE DISLOCATION

Fracture +/− dislocation of the tarsometatarsal (Lisfranc) joint of the foot. The injury takes its name from a Napoleonic surgeon who amputated feet at this point following trauma – often cavalrymen falling from and being dragged by their horse with foot still in the stirrup.

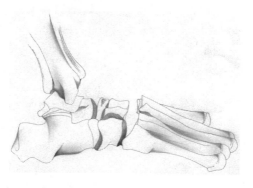

MAISONNEUVE'S FRACTURE

A proximal fibular fracture with distal tibiofibular syndesmosis rupture and medial or deltoid ligament injury or medial malleolar fracture.

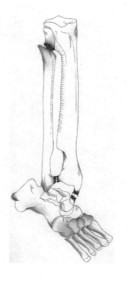

MALGAIGNE'S FRACTURE

An unstable pelvic fracture demonstrating vertical fracture lines anterior and posterior to the hip joint.

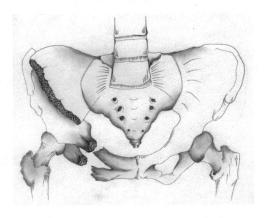

MALLET FINGER

A flexion deformity of the distal interphalangeal joint resulting from extensor tendon separation from the distal phalanx +/− avulsion of the dorsal lip of the phalanx. Often follows a forced flexion of the extended finger (e.g. mis-catching a ball), to rupture the extensor tendon or cause an avulsion fracture.

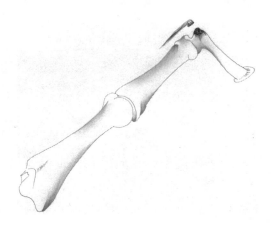

MONTEGGIA'S FRACTURE

A proximal third ulnar fracture with associated radial head dislocation, i.e. opposite to the Galleazi fracture.

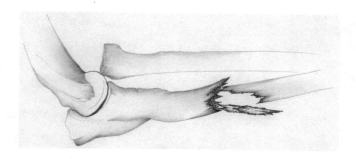

NIGHSTICK (PARRY) FRACTURE

An isolated mid-shaft ulnar fracture as a result of direct trauma, e.g. trying to defend against being hit by a weapon or item such as a police officer's truncheon or baton.

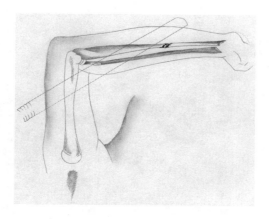

POTT'S FRACTURE

A distal fibular fracture 5–7.5 cm above the lateral malleolus with deltoid ligament rupture to allow lateral talar subluxation. Pott did not describe tibiofibular ligament disruption, which is often quoted.

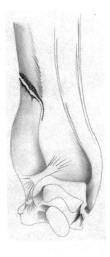

ROLANDO'S FRACTURE

A Y shaped intra articluar fracture of the base of the 1st metcarpal.

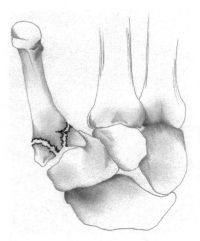

SEGOND'S FRACTURE

Avulsion fracture of the lateral tibial condyle at the iliotibial lip insertion point (Gurdey's tubercle). Strong association with internal derangement of the knee.

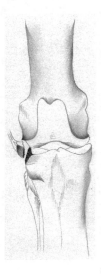

SHEPHERD'S FRACTURE

A fracture of the lateral tubercle of the posterior talar process.

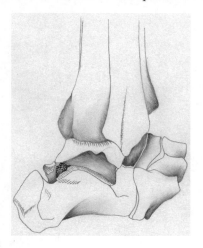

SMITH'S FRACTURE

A distal radial fracture with palmar displacement of the distal fracture fragment; also termed a reverse Colles fracture.

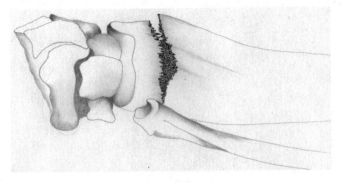

STIEDA'S (PELLIGRINI–STIEDA) FRACTURE

Avulsion of the medial femoral condyle at the origin of the medial femoral collateral ligament.

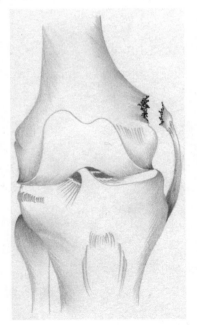

STRADDLE FRACTURE

Bilateral fractures of the superior and inferior pubic rami. May be noted in anterior compression injuries of the pelvis so should prompt a search for sacral or sacro-iliac injuries should a history suggest this mechanism.

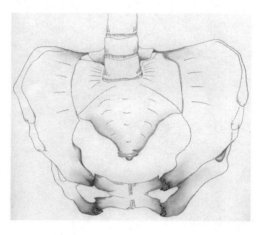

TEARDROP FRACTURE

A flexion fracture dislocation of the cervical spine to produce a triangular fracture fragment of the involved vertebrae. Due to posterior ligament disruption this injury is classified as unstable.

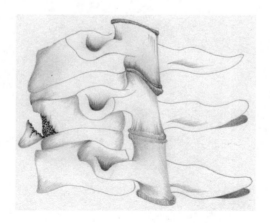

TILLAUX'S FRACTURE

Fracture of the lateral half of the distal tibial physis during closure as the skeleton matures. The medial half has usually fused.

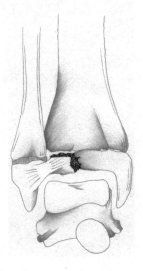

TORUS FRACTURE

A childhood impaction fracture causing buckling rather than complete fracture.

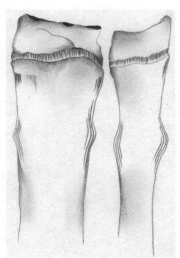

III Three-part where TWO segments are significantly displaced by more than 1 cm or angulated by 45°
IV Four-part where all FOUR major segments are displaced by 1 cm or angulated by 45°
V Fracture dislocation

Fractures of the distal clavicle

I Intact ligaments with no marked displacement
II Displaced interligamentous where the coracoclavicular ligaments detach from the medial segment and the trapezoid ligaments remain attached to the distal segment
III Fractures through the articular surface of the clavicle

HARRIS CLASSIFICATION

Cervical spine injuries

I Flexion (increasing severity/loss of stability)
   a Anterior subluxation
   b Bilateral interfacetal dislocation
   c Simple wedge compression fracture
   d Clay shoveller's fracture
   e Flexion teardrop
II Flexion Rotation – unilateral interfacetal dislocation
III Extension Rotation – pillar fracture
IV Vertical Compression
   a Jefferson burst fracture of C1
   b Burst fracture (remaining vertebral levels)
V Hyperextension (increasing severity or loss of stability)
   a Hyperextension dislocation
   b Avulsion of anterior arch of C1
   c Extension teardrop fracture of C2
   d Posterior arch fracture C1
   e Laminar fracture
   f Hangman's (traumatic spondylolisthesis) fracture
   g Hyperextension fracture dislocation
VI Lateral Flexion – uncinate process fracture
VII Varied Mechanisms
   a Atlanto-occipital dissociation
   b Odontoid fractures

ANDERSON AND D'ALONZO CLASSIFICATION

Odontoid peg fractures

I Oblique fracture through superior odontoid
II Fracture at junction between odontoid and body of axis
III Fracture at base of odontoid extending obliquely into body of
axis from posterior to anterior, superior to inferior

DENIS CLASSIFICATION

Thoracolumbar spinal injury

I Minor spinal injuries
   a Articular process fracture
   b Transverse process fracture
   c Spinous process fracture
   d Pars interarticularis fracture
II Major spinal injuries
   a Compression fracture
   b Burst fracture
   c Fracture dislocations
   d Seatbelt-type injuries

Sacral fractures

I Sacral ala fracture with no central canal or foramina damage
II Fracture involving sacral foramina, sparing the central canal
+/− fracture to the ala
III Fracture involving the central sacral canal +/− foramina
and ala

TILE CLASSIFICATION

Pelvic disruptions

Type A: stable
   A1 Pelvic fractures not involving the ring
   A2 Stable, minimally displaced fractures of the ring
Type B: rotationally unstable/vertically stable
   B1 Open book

B2 Lateral compression (ipsilateral)
B3 Lateral compression (contralateral) 'bucket handle' fractures

Type C: rotationally and vertically unstable
C1 Unilateral
C2 Bilateral
C3 Acetabular component

Acetabular fractures (displaced)
Type I: posterior fractures +/− posterior dislocation
A Posterior acetabular column
B Posterior acetabular wall
1 Associated with posterior column
2 Associated with transverse fractures
Type II: anterior fractures +/− anterior dislocation
A Anterior acetabular column
B Anterior acetabular wall
C Associated with anterior acetabular wall/column and/or transverse fractures
Type III: transverse types +/− central fracture dislocation
A Pure transverse
B T-shaped fractures
C Associated transverse and acetabular fractures
D Double column fractures

GARDEN CLASSIFICATION

Femoral neck fractures

I   Incomplete or impacted fracture
II Complete fracture but no displacement
III Complete fracture + partial displacement due to hip joint capsule being partially intact
IV Complete fracture + full displacement due to hip joint capsule being fully disrupted

KYLE CLASSIFICATION

Intertrochanteric hip fractures

I   Non-displaced, non-comminuted stable intertrochanteric fracture

II Displaced, minimally comminuted stable intertrochanteric fracture
III Displaced unstable intertrochanteric fracture demonstrating significant posteromedial comminution
IV Displaced unstable intertrochanteric fracture demonstrating significant posteromedial comminution + subtrochanteric component

AO CLASSIFICATION

Supracondylar femoral fractures
A Extra-articular
  A1 Avulsion of medial or lateral epicondyle
  A2 Simple supracondylar
  A3 Comminuted supracondylar
B Unicondylar
  B1 Medial or lateral condyle
  B2 Condyle fracture + extension into femoral shaft
  B3 Posterior tangential fracture of one or both condyles
C Bicondylar
  C1 Intercondylar
  C2 Intercondylar with a comminuted supracondylar component
  C3 Severely comminuted bicondylar fracture

Distal tibial (pilon) fractures

I A cleaving fracture (minus significant displacement) of the articular surface
II A cleaving fracture or the articular surface (minus extensive comminution) with significant articular incongruity
III A cleaving fracture of the articular surface + significant compression + displacement + comminution

Distal fibular fractures
A Transverse fracture of the fibula at or below the joint line
B Spiral fibular fracture beginning at the joint line + associated medial injury. Tibiofibular syndesmosis is intact though may be torn posteriorly
  C1 An oblique fibular fracture beginning above the ankle mortise. Tibiofibular syndesmosis is always disrupted as tibiofibular ligament is ruptured

C2 Oblique fibula fracture above ankle mortise with extensive tibiofibular syndesmosis disruption

LAUGE–HANSEN CLASSIFICATION

Ankle fractures (described by mechanism and/or resultant injury)

A Supination – eversion
  I   Anterior tibiofibular ligament disruption
  II   Spiral oblique fracture of distal fibula
  III Posterior tibiofibular ligament disrupted +/− posterior tibial lip fracture
  IV   Medial malleolar fracture/deltoid ligament tear
B Supination – adduction
  I   Transverse fracture of the lateral malleolus/rupture of collateral ligament
  II   Vertical fracture of medial malleolus
C Pronation – abduction
  I   Transverse fracture of the medial malleolus/deltoid ligament rupture
  II   Anterior and posterior tibiofibular ligament rupture +/− posterior margin fracture of tibia
  III Short horizontally directed oblique fracture of fibula
D Pronation – eversion
  I   Medial malleolar fracture/deltoid ligament rupture
  II   Anterior tibiofibular and interosseous ligament tear
  III Spiral fibular fracture 7–8 cm proximal to the tip of the lateral malleolus
  IV   Posterior tibial lip fracture
E Pronation – dorsiflexion
  I   Medial malleolar fracture/deltoid ligament rupture
  II   Anterior articular fracture of tibia due to talar dorsiflexed impaction
  III Supramalleolar fibular fracture
  IV   Avulsion of posterior tibia due to talar dorsiflexion and impaction

WEBER ANKLE FRACTURE CLASSIFICATION

Describes fractures of the lateral malleolus with respect to the level of the ankle joint. It is used to determine possible treatments.

Type A: Usually stable, there is a frequent fracture of the medial malleolus but the tibiofibular syndesmosis is intact, as is the deltoid ligament. The fracture is below the level of the ankle joint, making it stable. May require open reduction with internal fixation.

Type B: Usually begins at the level of the ankle joint. The fibular fracture extends superolaterally with the tibiofibular syndesmosis remaining intact or partly torn. There is no widening of the distal tibiofibular articulation. Stability varies according to presence of deltoid ligament tear of medial malleolar fracture.

Type C: Injury is above the level of the ankle joint with widening of the tibiofibular articulation due to tearing of the syndesmosis. There will be either a medial malleolus fracture or deltoid ligament tear. This is an unstable injury that will require open reduction with internal fixation.

Injuries and Classification Systems

Appendix 1

Common Radiological and Medical Abbreviations

?	Query
#	Fracture
<	Less than/below
>	More than/above
↑	Raised/hyper
↓	Lowered/hypo
2°	Secondary deposits (metastases)
AAA	Abdominal Aortic Aneurysm
Ab	Abortion of foetus
ABL	Anthropological Base Line
AC	Abdominal Circumference; AcromioClavicular; Alternating Current
ACJ	AcromioClavicular Joint
ACL	Anterior Cruciate Ligament
ACTH	AdrenoCorticoTrophic Hormone
ADE	Acute Demyelinating Encephalitis
ADH	AntiDiuretic Hormone
ADI	Acceptable Daily Intake
ADR	Adverse Drug Reaction
AE	After Evacuation
AF	Atrial Fibrillation
AFI	Amniotic Fluid Index
Ag	Antigen
AIDS	Acquired Immune Deficiency Syndrome
AIS	Adolescent Iodiopathic Scoliosis
AKA	Above-Knee Amputation; Also Known As
ALARA	As Low As Reasonably Achievable

ALARP	As Low As Reasonably Practicable
ALD	Alcoholic Liver Disease
ALL	Acute Lymphoblastic Leukaemia
ALLO	Atypical Legionella-Like Organisms
AM	After Micturition
AMI	Acute Myocardial Infarction
AML	Acute Myeloid Leukaemia
AP	AnteroPosterior
ARDS	Acute (Adult) Respiratory Distress Syndrome
ARF	Acute Renal Failure; Acute Respiratory Failure
ASD	Atrial Septal Defect
ASHD	ArterioSclerotic Heart Disease
ASIS	Anterior Superior Iliac Spine
ATN	Acute Tubular Necrosis
AVB	AtrioVentricular Block
AVH	Acute Viral Hepatitis
AVM	ArterioVenous Malformation
AVR	Aortic Valve Replacement
AXR	Abdominal X-Ray
Ba	Barium
$BaSO_4$	Barium Sulphate
BBB	Bundle Branch Block
BBV	Blood-Borne Virus
BE	Barium Enema
BEL	Breech, Extended Legs
BFL	Breech, Flexed Legs
BI	Bone Injury
BID	Brought In Dead (to hospital)
BIPAP	BiPhasic Positive Airways Pressure (ventilation)
BLS	Basic Life Support
BMD	Bone Mineral Density
BMI	Body Mass Index
BMR	Base Metabolic Rate
BMT	Bone Marrow Transplant
BO	Bowels Open
BOLD	Blood Oxygen Level Dependent
BPD	BiParietal Diameter
BPI	Blood Pressure Index
bpm	beats per minute
BSE	Bovine Spongiform Encephalopathy

BSR	Blood Sedimentation Rate
Bq	Bequerel
Ca	Carcinoma; Calcium
Ca^{2+}	Calcification
C_2H_5OH	inebriated with alcohol
CABG	Coronary Artery Bypass Graft
CAD	Coronary Artery Disease; Computer Aided Detection/Diagnosis
CAPD	Continuous Ambulatory Peritoneal Dialysis
CAT	Computed Axial Tomography
CBD	Common Bile Duct
CBF	Cerebral Blood Flow
CBP	Chronic Back Pain
CC	CranioCaudal
CCF	Congestive Cardiac Failure
CCU	Coronary Care Unit
CDH	Congenital Dislocation/Dysplasia of the Hip
CD-ROM	Compact Disc Read Only Memory
CD-RW	Compact Disc Read Write (Recordable)
CE FAST	Contrast-Enhanced Fourier-Acquired Steady sTate
CF	Cystic Fibrosis
CHD	Coronary Heart Disease
CHF	Congestive Heart Failure
CIBD	Chronic Inflammatory Bowel Disease
CJD	Creutzfeldt-Jakob Disease
CLL	Chronic Lymphocytic Leukaemia
CML	Chronic Myeloid Leukaemia
CNR	Contrast to Noise Ratio
C/O	Complains Of
CO(CI)	Cardiac Output (Cardiac Index)
COAD	Chronic Obstructive Airways Disease
COPD	Chronic Obstructive Pulmonary Disease
CP	Cerebral Palsy
CPAP(V)	Continuous Positive Airways Pressure (Ventilation)
CPB	CardioPulmonary Bypass
CPR	CardioPulmonary Resuscitation
CR	Computed Radiography
CRF	Chronic Renal Failure

CRL	Crown Rump Length
CSE	Conventional Spin Echo
CSF	CerebroSpinal Fluid
CT	Computed Tomography
CVA	CerebroVascular Accident
CVP	Central Venous Pressure
CVS	Chorionic Villus Sampling
CVVH(D)	Continuous Veno-Venous Haemo(dia)filtration (Haemodialysis)
CXR	Chest X-Ray
DCIS	Ductal Carcinoma In Situ
DDH	Developmental Dysplasia of Hip
DDR	Direct Digital Radiography
DE prep	Driven Equilibrium magnetisation *prep*aration
DEXA	Dual Energy X-ray Absorptiometry (DXA)
DIPJ	Distal InterPhalangeal Joint
DISH	Diffuse Idiopathic Skeletal Hyperostosis
DM	Diabetes Mellitus
DOA	Dead On Arrival
DP	dorsipalmar
DR	Digital Radiography
DRR	Digitally Reconstructed Radiographs
DRUJ	Distal RadioUlnar Joint
DVT	Deep Vein Thrombosis
DWI	Diffusion Weighted Imaging
Dx	Diagnosis
DDx	Differential Diagnosis
DXRT	Deep X-Ray Therapy
EAM	External Auditory Meatus
ECG	ElectroCardioGram
EDD	Expected Delivery Date
EDH	Extra(Epi)Dural Haemorrhage
EEG	ElectroEncephaloGram
EMI	Elderly with Mental Illness
ENT	Ear, Nose and Throat
Ep	Epilepsy
EPI	Echo Planar Imaging
ERCP	Endoscopic Retrograde Cholangio Pancreatography

E short	Short repetition technique based on echo
ESR	Erythrocyte Sedimentation Rate
ETOH	Inebriated with Ethanol (alcohol)
ETL	Echo Train Length
ETT	EndoTracheal Tube
EUA	Examination Under Anaesthetic
FAST	Fourier-Acquired Steady sTate
FAT SAT	Fat Saturation
FB	Foreign Body
FC	Flow Compensation
FFD	Fixed Flexion Deformity; Focus to Film Distance
FFE	Fast Field Echo
FH	Family History
FHR	Foetal Heart rate
FID	Focus to Image Distance; Free Induction Decay signal
FISP	Fast Imaging with Steady Precession
FL	Femur Length
FLAG	Flow-Adjusted Gradient
FLAIR	Fluid-Attenuated Inversion Recovery
FLASH	Fast Low-Angled Shot
FMNF	Foetal Movements Not Felt
fMRI	functional Magnetic Resonance Imaging
FN	False Negative
FNA(C)	Fine Needle Aspiration (Cytology)
FO	FrontoOccipital
FOV	Field Of View
FP	False Positive
FREEZE	Respiratory selection of phase-encoding steps
FSD	Focus to Skin Distance
FSE	Fast Spin Echo
F short	Short repetition technique based on free induction decay
FT	FollowThrough (small bowel imaging)
GA	General Anaesthetic
GBS	Guillain-Barré Syndrome
Gd	Gadolinium
Gd_2O_2S	Gadolinium Oxysulphide
$Gd_2O_2S.Tb$	Gadolinium Oxysulphide with Terbium activator

GFE	Gradient Field Echo
GFEC	Gradient Field Echo with Contrast
GFR	Glomerular Filtration Rate
GHRF	Growth Hormone Releasing Factor
GHIF	Growth Hormone Inhibiting Factor
GOO	Gastric Outlet Obstruction
GOR	Gastro-Oesophageal Reflux
GIT	GastroIntestinal Tract
GMN	Gradient Moment Nulling
GMR	Gradient Moment Rephasing
GR	Gradient Rephasing
GRASS	Gradient-Recalled Acquisition in the Steady State
GRE	Gradient Echo
GRE-EPI	Gradient Echo – Echo Planar Imaging
GTV	Gross Tumour Volume
GU	Gastric Ulcer; GenitoUrinary
GUM	GenitoUrinary Medicine
Gy	Gray

HAI	Hospital-Acquired Infection
HASTE	Half Acquisition Single shot Turbo spin Echo
Hb	Haemoglobin
HC	Head Circumference
HDU	High Dependency Unit
HGH	Human Growth Hormone
HI	Head Injury
HIS	Hospital Information System
HOCM	Hypertrophic Obstructive CardioMyopathy (HCM); High Osmolar Contrast Medium
HPC	History of Present Complaint
HPOA	Hypertrophic Pulmonary OsteoArthropathy
HRCT	High Resolution Computed Tomography
HRT	Hormone Replacement Therapy
HU	Hounsfield Units
HVL	Half Value Layer
Hx	History of …

IAM	Internal Auditory Meatus
IBD	Inflammatory Bowel Disease
IBS	Irritable Bowel Syndrome
ICP	Intra Cranial Pressure

ICRP	International Commission on Radiological Protection
ICU	Intensive Care Unit
IDDM	Insulin-Dependent Diabetes Mellitus
IDK	Internal Derangement of Knee
IF	Internal Fixation
Ig	Immunoglobulin
IHD	Ischaemic Heart Disease
IMRT	Intensity Modulated RadioTherapy
IOFB	IntraOrbital Foreign Body
IOL	Interorbital Line
IOML	InfraOrbitoMeatal Line
IOP	IntraOcular Pressure
IORT	IntraOperative RadioTherapy
IPH	IntraPartum Haemorrhage
IPL	InterPupillary Line
IPPV	Intermittent Positive Pressure Ventilation
IR	Inversion Recovery
IR-FSE	Inversion Recovery – Fast Spin Echo
IR prep	Inversion Recovery magnetisation preparation
ISD	Interventricular Septal Defect
IUCD	IntraUterine Contraceptive Device
IUD	IntraUterine Death; IntraUterine Device
IVC	Inferior Vena Cava
IVD	InterVertebral Disc
IVF	In Vitro Fertilisation
IVP	IntraVenous Pyelogram
IVU	IntraVenous Urogram
JCA	Juvenile Chronic Arthritis
JIS	Juvenile Idiopathic Scoliosis
KUB	Kidneys, Ureter and Bladder
LA	Left Atrium (Auricle)
LABC	Locally Advanced Breast Cancer
LAO	Left Anterior Oblique
LAN	Local Area Network
LAT	Lateral
LBP	Low Back Pain
LCIS	Lobular Carcinoma In Situ

Appendix 1

LCM	Lower Costal Margin
LFT	Liver Function Test
LIF	Left Iliac Fossa
LIMA	Left Internal Mammary Artery
LLL	Left Lower Lobe (of the lung)
LLO	Legionella-Like Organism
LMP	Last Menstrual Period
LOCM	Low Osmolar Contrast Medium
LPO	Left Posterior Oblique
LRTI	Lower Respiratory Tract Infection
LUL	Left Upper Lobe
LV	Left Ventricle
LVF	Left Ventricular Failure
MABP	Mean Arterial Blood Pressure
MAST	Motion Artefact Suppression
MC	MetaCarpal
MCP	MetaCarpoPhalangeal
MCPJ	MetaCarpoPhalangeal Joint
MDR-TB	Multiple Drug Resistant TuBerculosis
MEMP	Multi Echo Multi Planar
MI	Mitral Incompetence/Insufficiency; Myocardial Infarction
MIPS	Maximum Intensity ProjectionS
MPAP	Mean Pulmonary Artery Pressure
MPD	Maximum Permissible Dose
MPGR	MultiPlanar Gradient-Recalled acquisition in the steady state
MPIR	MultiPlanar Inversion Recovery
MPR	MultiPlanar Reconstruction
MP RAGE	Magnetisation Prepared RApid Gradient Echo
MR	Mitral Regurgitation; Magnetic Resonance
MRA	Magnetic Resonance Angiography
MRCP	Magnetic Resonance Cholangio Pancreatography
MRI	Magnetic Resonance Imaging
MRSA	Meticillin-Resistant *Staphylococcus Aureus*
MS	Mitral Stenosis; Multiple Sclerosis
MSP	Mid-/Median Sagittal Plane; Munchausen Syndrome by Proxy
MSU	MidStream Urine
MT	Magnetisation Transfer; Metatarsal

MTP	MetaTarsoPhalangeal
MTPJ	MetaTarsoPhalangeal Joint
MVA	Motor Vehicle Accident
MVD	Mitral Valve Disease
MVR	Mitral Valve Replacement
Mx	Mastectomy
Mz	Longitudinal Magnetisation
NAD	No Abnormality Detected
NAI	Non-Accidental Injury
NAR	Nasal Airway Resistance
NB	Nota Bene (take note)
NBI	No Bone Injury
NBM	Nil By Mouth
NFS	No Fracture Seen/Shown
NG	NasoGastric; New Growth
NGT	NasoGastric Tube
NHL	Non Hodgkin's Lymphoma
NICU	Neonatal Intensive Care Unit
NIPPV	Non-invasive Intermittent Positive Pressure Ventilation
NM	Nuclear Medicine
NMR	Nuclear Magnetic Resonance
NND	NeoNatal Death
NPV	Negative Predictive Value
NRDS	Neonatal Respiratory Distress Syndrome
NSAIDs	NonSteroidal Anti-Inflammatory Drugs
NSCLC	Non Small-Cell Lung Cancer
NSU	Non-Specific Urethritis
NWB	Non Weight-Bearing
O_2	Oxygen
OA	OsteoArthritis
OC	Oral Contraceptive
OD	OverDose
OE	On Examination
OF	OccipitoFrontal
OHS	Open Heart Surgery
OM	OccipitoMental
OMBL	OrbitoMeatal Base Line
OML	OrbitoMeatal Line

OR	Open Reduction
ORIF	Open Reduction (with) Internal Fixation
OT	Occupational Therapist; Operating Theatre
PA	Pernicious Anaemia; PosteroAnterior
PAFC	Pulmonary Artery Flotation Catheter
PC	Phase Contrast
PC-MRA	Phase Contrast Magnetic Resonance Angiography
PCL	Posterior Cruciate Ligament
PCTA	PerCutaneous Transluminal Angioplasty
PD	Proton Density
PDA	Patent Ductus Arteriosus
PE	Pulmonary Embolism
PEAR	Phase-Encoding Artefact Reduction
PET	Positron Emission Tomography
PFO	Patent Foramen Ovale
PID	Prolapsed Intervertebral Disc; Pelvic Inflammatory Disease
PIH	Pregnancy-Induced Hypertension
PIP	Proximal InterPhalangeal
PIPJ	Proximal InterPhalangeal Joint
PM	Post Micturition; Post Mortem
PNS	PostNasal Space
POM	Prescription Only Medicine
PoP	Plaster Of Paris
PPV	Positive Predictive Value
PR	Per Rectum
PRF	Pulse Repetition Frequency
PSA	Prostate-Specific Antigen
PSIS	Posterior Superior Iliac Spine
PTB	Pulmonary TuBerculosis
PTC	Percutaneous Transhepatic Cholangiogram
PTE	Pulmonary ThromboEmbolism
PTRF	Post Transplant Renal Failure
PTV	Planning Target Volume
PU	Passed Urine; Peptic Ulcer
PUO	Pyrexia of Unknown Origin
PTX	PneumoThoraX
PV	Per Vaginam
PWB	Partial Weight Bearing
Px	Prognosis; Pneumothorax

Appendix 1

QA	Quality Assurance
QALYs	Quality Adjusted Life Years
QoL	Quality of Life
RA	Rheumatoid Arthritis; Right Atrium (Auricle)
RAM FAST	Rapid Acquisition Matrix FAST (Fourier-Acquired Steady sTate)
RAO	Right Anterior Oblique
RAS	Renal Artery Stenosis
RB	Recurrent Bleed
RBBB	Right Bundle Branch Block
RBC	Red Blood Cell
RBL	Radiographic Base Line
RCR	Royal College of Radiologists
RCT	Randomised Controlled Trial
RDS	Respiratory Distress Syndrome; Red Dot System
REST	Regional Saturation Technique
RF	Radio Frequency
RHD	Rheumatic Heart Disease
RICE	Rest, Ice, Compression, Elevation
RICP	Raised IntraCranial Pressure (RIP)
RIF	Right Iliac Fossa
RIS	Radiology Information System
RLL	Right Lower Lobe (of lung)
RML	Right Middle Lobe (of lung)
RNI	RadioNuclide Imaging
ROC	Receiver Operator Characteristic
ROI	Region Of Interest
ROM	Range Of Movement
RPN	Renal Papillary Necrosis
RPO	Right Posterior Oblique
RSI	Repetitive Strain Injury
RTA	Road Traffic Accident
RTP	Radiation Treatment Planning
RUL	Right Upper Lobe (of lung)
RV	Right Ventricle
Rx	Therapy
SAH	SubArachnoid Haemorrhage
SARA	Sexually Acquired Reactive Arthritis
SAT	Saturation

SCBU	Special Care Baby Unit
SCC	Spinal Cord Compression; Squamous Cell Carcinoma
SCLC	Small Cell Lung Cancer
SCJ	SternoClavicular Joint
SDH	SubDural Haemorrhage/Haematoma
SE	Spin Echo; Standard Error
SE-EPI	Spin Echo – Echo Planar Imaging
Short	Short repetition techniques
SID	Source to Image Distance
SIDS	Sudden Infant Death Syndrome (cot death)
SIJ	Sacro-Iliac Joint
SHO	Senior House Officer (Junior grade doctor)
SLD	SubLethal Damage
SLDR	SubLethal Damage Recovery
SMART	Sterotactic Multiple Arc RadioTherapy
SMASH	Short Minimum Angled SHot
SMR	Standardised Mortality Ratio; SubMucous Resection
SMV	SubMento Vertex (Vertical)
SNR	Signal to Noise Ratio
SOB	Short Of Breath
SOBOE	Shortness Of Breath On Exertion
SOL	Space-Occupying Lesion
SPAMM	SPAtial Modulation of Magnetisation
SPECT	Single Photon Emission Computed Tomography
SPGR	Spoiled GRASS
SPIR	SPectrally selective Inversion Recovery
SS	Single Shot
SSD	Source to Skin Distance
SS-EPI	Single Shot – Echo Planar Imaging
SSFP	Steady State Free Precession
SS-FSE	Single Shot – Fast Spin Echo
STAGE	Small Tip Angle Gradient Echo
STD	Sexually Transmitted Disease
STERF	Steady state TEchnique with Refocused Free Induction Decay
STI	Sexually Transmitted Infection
STIR	Short T1 Inversion Recovery
Sv	Sievert
SV	Stroke Volume

SVC	Superior Vena Cava
SXR	Skull X-Ray
T1	Longitudinal magnetisation relaxation time
T2	Transverse magnetisation relaxation time
T21	Trisomy 21 (Down syndrome)
TAUS	TransAbdominal UltraSound
TB	TuBerculosis
TBI	Total Body Irradiation
TDF	Time, Dose, Fractionation
TE	Time to Echo
TFE	Turbo Field Echo
THR	Total Hip Replacement
TI	Time to Inversion
TIA	Transient Ischaemic Attack
TIPSS	Transjugular Intrahepatic PortoSystemic Shunting
TKR	Total Knee Replacement
TLD	ThermoLuminescent Dosimeter
TMJ	TemporoMandibular Joint
TN	True Negative
TNF	Tumour Necrosis Factor
TNM	Tumour (lymph) Node Metastasis
TOE	TransOesophageal Echo
TOF	Time Of Flight; Tetralogy Of Fallot; Tracheo-Oesophageal Fistula
TOF-MRA	Time Of Flight–Magnetic Resonance Angiography
TOP	Termination Of Pregnancy
TP	Terminal Phalanx; True Positive
TPR	Temperature, Pulse, Respiration
TR	Repetition Time
TRUS	TransRectal UltraSound
TSE	Turbo Spin Echo
TSS	Toxic Shock Syndrome
TURP	TransUrethral Resection of Prostate
TVUS	TransVaginal UltraSound
Tx	Transplant; Treatment; Therapy
UNSCEAR	United Nations Scientific Committee on the Effects of Atomic Radiation
URTI	Upper Respiratory Tract Infection
US	UltraSound

USB	Universal Serial Bus
UTI	Urinary Tract Infection
VDU	Visual Display Unit
VEB	Ventricular Ectopic Beats
VEMP	Variable Echo MultiPlanar
VENC	Velocity ENCoding
VLBW	Very Low Birth Weight
V/Q	Ventilation/Perfusion ratio
VSD	Ventricular Septal Defect
WAN	Wide Area Network
WB	Weight Bearing
WBC	White Blood Cell
WBCC	White Blood Cell Count
WG	Wegener's Granuloma
WHO	World Health Organization
W_T	Tissue Weighting factor

Appendix 2

Glossary of Common Terms for Medical Radiation Practice (including prefixes and suffixes)

a	prefix – without/absence of
ab	prefix – away from
abdomin	prefix – abdomen
abortion	natural or artificial expulsion of the foetus/embryo from the uterus
ac	suffix – pertaining to
acetabul	prefix – acetabulum
acou	prefix – hearing
abscess	localised collection of pus
achalasia	obstruction caused by non-relaxed muscular layer/sphincter
achondroplasia	failure of endochondral ossification to cause dwarfism
acoustic neuroma	benign tumour found on eighth cranial nerve
acromegaly	overgrowth of soft and bony tissues due to a pituitary tumour
ad	prefix – to or toward
Addison's disease	chronic adrenal cortical failure noted in adults
aden	prefix – gland
adenoma	benign glandular tissue tumour
adhesions	fibrous tissue bands from surgical or inflammatory causes
adren	prefix – adrenal gland
aemia	suffix – of the blood

Index of Medical Imaging, First Edition. Jonathan McConnell.
© 2011 Blackwell Publishing Ltd. Published 2011 by Blackwell Publishing Ltd.

aer	prefix – air or gas
agra	suffix – extreme pain
akathisia	inability to remain motionless, as seen in Parkinson's disease, or a feeling of inner restlessness
al	suffix – relating to
albuminuria	urine containing albumin
algesi	prefix – pain
algia	suffix – pain
alopecia	loss of hair
Alport's syndrome	albuminuria plus deafness and eye lesions
aluminosis	lung fibrosis caused by metallic dust inhalation
amenorrhoea	absence of the menstrual periods
amni	prefix – amnion
amyl	prefix – starch
an	prefix – without or absence of
andr	prefix – male
anencephaly	congenital absence of the cranial vault and brain
aneurysm	distension of a duct or artery of a localised nature
angio	prefix – vessel
angioma	benign tumour of blood vessel association
anis	prefix – unequal
ankyl	prefix – crooked, stiff or bent
ankylosing spondylitis	inflammatory arthritic process of the spine causing vertebral fusion
ankylosis	immobilisation of a joint
ante	prefix – before
antepartum	before delivery of a child
anti	prefix – against
antr	prefix – antrum
anu	prefix – anus
aort	prefix – aorta
aortic regurgitation	backflow of blood through the aortic valve of the heart
aortic stenosis	an abnormal narrowing of the aortic valve

apheresis	suffix – removal
apo	prefix – upon
aponeur	prefix – aponeurosis
appendic	prefix – appendix
ar	suffix – relating to
arachno	prefix – spider-like
arachnodactyly	'spider digits' or abnormally long fingers or toes
arche	prefix – first or beginning
areflexia	absence of the reflexes
arteri	prefix – artery
arteriosclerosis	artery hardening with accompanying narrowing of the vessel lumen
arthr	prefix – joint
arthrodesis	surgical fusion of a joint
articul	prefix – joint
ary	suffix – relating to
asbestosis	lung disease due to dust (asbestos)
ascites	excess intraperitoneal fluid
ase	suffix – enzyme
asthenia	suffix – generalised nonspecific weakness
astrocytoma	cranial tumour – commonest form of glioma
atel	prefix – incomplete or imperfect
atelectasis	non-expansion or partial collapse of the lung
ather	prefix – yellow fatty blood vessel plaque
atheroma	fatty layering/degenerative change of the lining of blood vessels, usually arterial
atherosclerosis	arterial disease with atheroma
atresia	the normal lumen of hollow organs fails to develop
atrophy	abnormal reduction in the size of tissues
aur	prefix – ear
auricular fibrillation	abnormality in the heart rhythm
avulsion	plucking away or tearing off of bone fragment at a tendon or ligament insertion
axill	prefix – armpit

benign	non-malignant or simple tumour
Bennett's fracture	two-part intra-articular fracture of the base of the first metacarpal
bi	prefix – two
bil	prefix – bile or biliary
blast	prefix – developing cell, e.g. blastocyst, or Suffix as in osteoblast
brachi	prefix – arm
brachycephaly	caused by premature suture closure to create a short high skull
brady	prefix – slow
Bright's disease	renal pathology – a form of nephritis
bronch	prefix – bronchus
bronchiectasis	bronchial dilation, often following an infection
bucc	prefix – cheek, e.g. buccal cavity = mouth
burs	prefix – bursa, a type of sac or cavity
bursa	fluid-filled pocket-like structure often associated with a joint
bursitis	inflammation of a bursa
calc	prefix – calcium
calculus	a stone or rounded calcific density
callus	a collar of extra bone found during the fracture healing process
capnia	suffix – content of carbon dioxide in the blood (excess = hypercapnia)
carcin	prefix – cancer
carcinoma	malignant tumour (cancer) from epithelial tissue
carcinomatosis	The spread of a carcinoma (secondaries, metastases)
cardi	prefix – heart
carditis	heart inflammation
carp	prefix – carpal bones
cata	prefix – down/reduced, e.g. catatonic = reduced motor skills
caud	prefix – caudal or toward the tail or lower part of the body
cellulitis	dispersed infection of connective tissue

centesis	suffix – surgical puncture to aspirate fluid, e.g. amniocentesis
ceph	prefix – head or toward the head or upper part of the body
cerebell	prefix – cerebellum
cerebr	prefix – cerebrum or main hemispheres of the brain
chol	prefix – bile or linked to biliary system
cholangi	prefix – bile ducts
cholangitis	inflammation of the biliary ducts
cholecystectomy	surgical removal of the gallbladder
cholecystitis	gallbladder inflammation
choledoch	prefix – common bile duct
choledocholithiasis	condition of the presence of calculi in the common bile duct
cholelithiasis	stone formation in the gall bladder or biliary ducts, may be calcific or cholesterol in nature
chondr	prefix – cartilage
chondroma	a benign cartilaginous tumour
chondromalacia patellae	a softening of the chondral cartilage on the posterior surface of the patella, resulting in pain and reduced mobility
chordoma	uncommon locally malignant skull or sacral tumour
chori	prefix – chorion
chrom	prefix – colour
cidal	suffix – killing (to kill)
clasia	suffix – break (clasis and clast)
claudication	reduced blood supply to the muscle, results in pain on exertion
clavic	prefix – pertaining to the clavicle
clysis	suffix – irrigate or wash
coarctation	a congenital narrowing of the thoracic aorta
coccus	suffix – berry-shaped bacterium (pl. cocci)
coeliac disease	malabsorption due dietary gluten sensitivity that causes loss of intestinal villi

col	prefix – colon related
colp	prefix – vagina
con	prefix – together
congenital	present at birth
congestion	a build-up of excess fluid in the body tissues, noted particularly in the air spaces of the lungs
coni	related to dust, e.g. pneumoconiosis
consolidation	when exudate in the lungs solidifies
contra	prefix – opposite, e.g. contralateral = on the opposite side
contusion	bruising
coron	prefix – heart related, e.g. coronary artery
cortc	prefix – cortex, e.g. cortical margin of the radius
cost	prefix – rib (costo)
coxa vara	congenital malformation of the femoral neck to generate excessive angulation toward the midline
crani	prefix – skull
craniostenosis	premature closure of the sutures of the skull bones
crepitus	that sound and feeling of the ends of a fracture or joint surfaces rubbing together, or breath sounds in the lungs from a range of respiratory diseases
crit	suffix – to separate
Crohn's disease	chronic nonspecific inflammation of any part of the intestine though linked more frequently with the small bowel
croup	an infant's cough with associated dyspnoea due to mucosal swelling
Cushing's syndrome	the effect of excessive adrenal corticosteroids
cyanosis	blue tinge of the skin that is due to insufficient oxygenation
cyst	a sac that contains fluid or semi-solid material, e.g. pus or fat

cyto	prefix – cell
cyte	suffix – cell
dacry	prefix – tear or tear duct
dacryoadenitis	lacrimal gland inflammation
dactyl	prefix – fingers or toes
degloving	detachment of the skin from underlying tissues as a result of trauma
dent	prefix – tooth
derm	prefix – skin
dermoid cyst	a benign cystic teratoma of mature skin that may contain a collection of sebum, nails, hair, teeth, eyes, cartilage and thyroid tissue
desis	suffix – surgical fusion or fixation, e.g. arthrodesis
dextr	prefix – right
dextrocardia	the heart is situated on the right side of the thorax (situs inversus = mirror image of normal arrangement)
diabetes mellitus	high blood sugar due to insufficient insulin production or the body's failure to respond to insulin
diaphysis	the shaft of a long bone
dis	prefix – to free from or undo
dislocation	complete displacement of the alignment of bones that form a joint
distal	prefix – furthest away from the centre
diverticulitis	inflammation of the diverticulae of the bowel
diverticulosis	the condition of having multiple bowel diverticulae
diverticulum	an abnormal outpouching from a hollow organ, e.g. large bowel
dors	prefix – back of the body
duoden	prefix – relating to duodenum
dys	prefix – abnormal, painful, difficult or laboured
dysmenorrhoea	painful menstrual periods

Appendix 2

dyspepsia	indigestion
dysphagia	difficulty in swallowing
dysphasia	speech impediment caused by cerebral cortical insufficiency such as following a stroke
dysplasia	abnormality of growth of a tissue
dyspnoea	difficulty in breathing
dystrophy	abnormal development of a tissue, most common associations are muscle and bone that may be linked to other disease, e.g. renal osteodystrophy
dysuria	painful and difficult micturition
eal	suffix – pertaining to, e.g. epiphyseal
ectasis	suffix – to stretch, expand or dilate
ecto	prefix – outside or outer
ectomy	suffix – excision or surgical removal
ectop	prefix – located away from the usual place
ectopia	suffix – displacement
ectopic pregnancy	when the foetus implants and forms outside the uterus
effusion	fluid formation within a body cavity
ema	suffix – swelling
embolism	obstruction of blood flow to a structure by a clot or other material, e.g. fat or air
emesis	suffix – vomiting
emia	suffix – condition of the blood
emphysema	a chronic lung disease where the alveoli break down to form larger air spaces and reduce gaseous exchange efficiency. Emphysema may also be surgical where gas leaks into tissues such as follow the insertion of an intrathoracic drain for other conditions and is visible radiographically
empyema	a collection of pus within a naturally occurring cavity, e.g. pleura of the lung

encephal	prefix – relating to the brain
encephalitis	inflammation of the brain
enchondroma	benign cartilaginous tumour growing inside the bone
endo	prefix – within or inner
endocarditis	inflammation of the heart's endocardium
enter	prefix – relating to the intestines
enteritis	intestinal inflammation of a regional nature
enuresis	incontinence of urine
epi	prefix – on, upon or over
epididym	prefix – relating to the epididymis
epiglott	prefix – relating to the epiglottis
epilepsy	an episodic brain disorder resulting in a fit or seizure
episi	prefix – relating to the vulva, e.g. episiotomy during childbirth
epistaxis	nose bleed
epitheli	prefix – epithelium
epithelioma	tumour of the epithelial cells
erythr	prefix – red, as in erythrocytes or red blood cells
esis	suffix – condition
esophago	prefix – relating to oesophagus
esthesi	sensation, feeling or sensitivity, e.g. anaesthesia
etio	prefix – cause of a disease
Ewing's sarcoma	a small cell carcinoma of juvenile bones
ex	prefix – outside
exacerbation	an increase in severity
exostosis	a bony outgrowth
extra	prefix – beyond or outside
faci	prefix – related to face
femor	prefix – related to femur
fferent	suffix – to carry, e.g. afferent vessels
fibr	prefix – fibrous tissues
fibrillation	rapid and irregular muscle movement
fibroid	a simple uterine tumour
fistula	an abnormal communication between structures or organs

flail chest	multiple fractures of the ribs that produces paradoxical ventilation of the chest
Freiberg's disease	aseptic necrosis of the second (usual) or other metatarsal head
Galeazzi's fracture dislocation	a fracture of the mid to distal third of the radius with dislocation of the distal radioulnar joint
gangrene	tissue necrosis due to lack of blood supply/oxygenation
gastro	prefix – stomach
gen	suffix – substance, agent, object that causes, e.g. pathogen
genesis	suffix – cause or beginning/origin
genic	suffix – producing, generating, causing, originating
ger	prefix – old age
geront	prefix – old age
gingiv	prefix – pertaining to the gums
glioma	general term for a nervous system tumour
globin	suffix – a type of protein, e.g. haemoglobin
glomerul	prefix – pertaining to the glomerulus (of the kidney)
gloss	prefix – relating to the tongue
gluc	prefix – sugar
glyc	prefix – sugar
glycosuria	sugar in the urine
gnath	prefix – relating to the jaw
gnos	prefix – knowledge of
goitre	an enlargement of the thyroid gland
gout	due to excess uric acid in the blood – linked to arthritic changes
grand mal	epilepsy with classical fitting episodes – now termed tonic-clonic seizure
gravid	prefix – pregnancy, pregnant woman
greenstick fracture	bending of one bone cortex with splitting fracture of opposite cortex in juvenile bones

Appendix 2

Guillain-Barré syndrome	acute disorder with loss of peripheral nerve conduction and associated respiratory difficulty
gynae	prefix – woman
haem	prefix – the blood
haemangioma	tumour of vascular tissue
haematemesis	vomiting of blood
haematuria	blood in the urine
haemoptysis	coughing up of blood
hallux valgus	deviation of the big toe to towards the little toe. The first metatarsal also deviates toward the midline – may generate a bunion at the metatarsophalangeal joint
hemi	prefix – one half
hemiplegia	paralysis of one side of the body
hepat	prefix – pertaining to the liver
hepatitis	inflammation of the liver
hernia	abnormal protrusion of tissue through an orifice
heter	prefix – other
hiatus hernia	protrusion of an abdominal organ (often stomach) through the diaphragm
hidr	prefix – pertaining to sweat
Hirschsprung's disease	congenital absence of nervous supply to a portion of the colon so that there is dilation and hypertrophy of the large bowel to cause an obstruction
hist	prefix – pertaining to tissue
Hodgkin's disease	a cancer of the lymphocytes to affect the lymphatic system
hom	prefix – same
hydatid cyst	a cyst formed by tapeworm infestation of the *Echinococcus* genus
hydr	prefix – pertaining to water
hydrocephalus	excess cerebrospinal fluid in the cranial vault

Appendix 2

hydronephrosis	kidney enlargement due to obstruction
hydropneumothorax	the presence of fluid and air in the pleural cavity
hydrothorax	fluid in the pleural cavity often from liver cirrhosis or ascites
hyper	prefix – above or excessive
hyperglycaemia	excess sugar in the bloodstream
hypernephroma	cancer of the renal parenchymal tissues
hyperplasia	tissue enlargement without new growth
hypertension	abnormally high blood pressure
hypertrophy	organ enlargement through increased use
hypn	prefix – relating to sleep
hypo	prefix – below, less than, incomplete
hypoplasia	underdevelopment
hyster	prefix – relating to the uterus
ia	suffix – abnormal or diseased state
ial	suffix – pertaining to
iasis	suffix – tends to form or condition, e.g. urolithiasis
iatr	prefix – physician or medicine
iatry	suffix – physician or treatment
ic	suffix – pertaining to
ician	suffix – one who, e.g. paediatrician
ictal	suffix – attach or seizure
idiopathic	describing a spontaneous disease of unknown cause
ile	prefix – relating to the ileum
ileitis	inflammation of the ileum
ileostomy	surgical opening of the ileum onto the abdominal wall
ileus	intestinal obstruction, usually linked to the small bowel
ili	prefix – relating to the ilium
immune	prefix – immune
in	prefix – in or into; not
infra	prefix – under or below
infarction	death of cells and tissues due to loss of blood supply

Appendix 2

inflammation	a local reaction to damage or infection of cells
inter	prefix – between
intra	prefix – within
intussussception	obstruction caused by invagination of the bowel into a more distal part, thus preventing normal peristalsis
iri(d)	prefix – iris
is	prefix – equal or the same as
isch	prefix – deficiency, e.g. ischaemia
ischaemia	local deficiency of blood supply
ism	suffix – having a condition
itis	suffix – inflammation
jaundice	skin yellowing from excessive bilirubin in the bloodstream
jejun	prefix – relating to the jejunum
juxta	prefix – adjacent to, e.g. juxta-articular
kal	prefix – relating to potassium
kary	prefix – nucleus, e.g. karyotype
Keinbock's disease	aseptic necrosis of the lunate
kerat	prefix – hard or horny tissue; cornea
kinesi	prefix – movement
Kippel–Feil syndrome	congenital short neck with vertebral fusion
Köhler's disease	aseptic necrosis of the navicular
kyph	prefix – hump
kyphosis	excessive concavity of the anterior of the spine, thoracic spine creates a 'hunchback' or 'dowager's hump'
labi	prefix – lips
lacrim	prefix – tear duct, tear related
lact	prefix – milk
lamin	prefix – pertaining to the lamina
laminectomy	surgical removal of the lamina of the vertebra to expose the spinal cord
lapar	prefix – abomen, e.g. laparotomy
laryng	prefix – pertaining to the larynx
later	prefix – side, e.g. lateral decubitus

lei	prefix – smooth, e.g. leiomyosarcoma
lepsy	suffix – seizure
lesion	any damage or injury that causes a change to tissue
leuk	prefix – white
leukaemia	malignant excessive production of white blood cells
lingu	prefix – pertaining to the tongue
lip	prefix – fat
lipoma	a fat-cell-based benign tumour
lith	stone, e.g. lithotomy
lob	prefix – pertaining to a lobe
lord	prefix – bent forward
lordosis	excessive anterior convexity of the spine
lumbago	localised pain emanating from the lumbar spine
lymph	prefix – pertaining to lymph
lymphoma	lymphoid tissue tumour (see Hodgkin's disease)
lysis	suffix – loosening, separating or dissolution, i.e. breaking down
lytic	suffix – destroy, breakdown or reduce, e.g. haemolytic enzymes
macro	prefix – large, magnified, wider, e.g. macroscopic
mal	prefix – bad
malacia	suffix – softening, e.g. osteomalacia
malaise	a generalised feeling of being unwell
malignant	describing a tumour that is life-threatening and usually produces secondary effects
mamm	prefix – pertaining to the breast
mast	prefix – relating to the breast
mastectomy	surgical removal of the breast
mastoidectomy	surgical removal of one of the mastoid air cells such as for tumour excision
maxill	prefix – pertaining to the maxilla
meat	prefix – opening, e.g. external auditory meatus

Meckel's diverticulum	a rudimentary duct that creates an outpouching of the ileal wall
megacolon	colonic dilation with constipation (see Hirschsprung's disease)
megaly	suffix – enlargement
melaena	blackening of the faeces by altered blood
melanoma	melanocyte (pigment-producing cells of the skin) tumour
Menière's disease	inner ear disease with linked tinnitus and vertigo
meninges	the three membranes that cover the brain and spinal cord
meningioma	usually benign tumour of the meninges that may calcify
meningitis	inflammation of the meninges
meningocoele	congenital herniation of the meninges through the skull or spinal cord
meniscectomy	surgical removal of the meniscal cartilage of the knee joint
menorrhagia	excessive blood loss during the menstrual periods
ment	prefix – pertaining to the mind, e.g. mental
meso	prefix – middle, e.g. mesoderm
meta	prefix – change, after, beyond, e.g. metastatic
metr	prefix – pertaining to the uterus, e.g. endometrium
metry	suffix – measurement
micro	prefix – small, e.g. microscopic
morph	prefix or Suffix – shape or form
muc	prefix – mucus
multi	prefix – many
multigravida	a woman with one or many previous pregnancies
multiparous	a woman who has given birth to more than one child
mumps	acute infection of the parotid salivary glands
my(o)	prefix – muscle

myc	prefix – fungus
myasthenia gravis	a disease that demonstrate voluntary muscle weakness
myel	prefix – spinal cord (i.e. nerve related) or bone marrow, e.g. myeloma
myeloma	a bone marrow tumour (plasmacytoma) that has many deposits throughout the skeleton
myocarditis	inflammation of the heart muscle
myositis ossificans	ossification of haematoma (or free blood) over a bone or joint following trauma or insufficient wound drainage after surgery
naevus	a well-circumscribed mole or birth mark of the skin
narc	prefix – stupor, e.g. narcotics
nas	prefix – pertaining to the nose
nat	prefix – birth
necr	prefix – death of cells or body (of tissue)
necrosis	death of an organ or tissues within a living body
neo	prefix – new
neoplasm	a tumour or new growth that may have benign or malignant properties
nephr	prefix – pertaining to the kidney
nephrectomy	surgical removal of a kidney
nephritis	inflammation of a kidney (or kidney parenchyma)
nephrostomy	surgical drainage of the kidney, may be performed in the radiology interventional suite
neuro	prefix – pertaining to the nervous system
neuralgia	nervous system pain, e.g. facial neuralgia
neuroblastoma	a malignant childhood tumour of the adrenal medullary tissue
neurofibroma	a benign tumour originating from the fibrous sheath of a nerve

Appendix 2

noct	prefix – night
nulli	prefix – none
nyct	prefix – night
nyctal	suffix – night
ocul	prefix – pertaining to the eye
odia	suffix – small
odynia	suffix – pain
oedema	fluid increase within tissues
oesophageal varices	dilation of lower oesophageal veins caused by redirection of the hepatic portal vein blood flow in the cirrhotic liver
oid	suffix – resembling
olig	prefix – few, e.g. oligaemia
ologist	suffix – a specialist in
ology	suffix – the science or study of
oma	suffix – swelling or tumour, e.g. osteoma
onc	prefix – tumour, e.g. oncology
orrhagia	suffix – rapid flow, e.g. haemorrhage
opth	prefix – pertaining to the eye
opthalm	prefix – eye
opia	suffix – condition, vision
opsy	suffix – to view, e.g. biopsy
or	prefix – pertaining to the mouth
orch	prefix – pertaining to the testicle or testis
orraphy	suffix – suture
orrhoea	suffix – excess flow
orrhexis	suffix – to rupture
orth	prefix – straight, correct, e.g. orthodontic
ory	suffix – referring to
oscopy	suffix – visualise using an endoscope
Osgood-Sclatter's disease	osteochondritis of the tibial tubercle often examined with ultrasound or MRI
osis	suffix – condition (having a condition), increased

Appendix 2

oste	prefix – pertaining to bone
osteitis	bone inflammation, e.g. osteitis pubis
osteoarthritis	degenerative arthritis of a chronic nature resulting in joint space loss, subchondral cysts and sclerosis plus osteophytosis
osteochondroma	a benign bone and cartilaginous tumour
osteoclastoma	also termed giant cell tumour. Massive local bone destruction that requires surgical removal and grafting. Often noted around the knee in the femur or tibia
osteogenesis imperfecta	congenitally defective connective tissue resulting in brittle bones
osteoma	benign skull or facial bone (commonly) tumour
osteomalacia	adult vitamin D deficiency resulting in ineffective mineralisation of osteoid tissue, termed rickets in children
osteomyelitis	bone (and associated soft tissue) inflammation as a result of infection that may be dormant for years of spread in the blood from a second infection site
osteopenia	a reduced bone density
osteopoikilosis	a benign bone variation that is characterised by multiple sclerotic 'spots', mainly metaphyseal in position
osteoporosis	loss of bone tissue with insufficient replacement of new material – measurable with DEXA or qualitative CT
ostomy	suffix – creating an opening, e.g. colostomy
ot	prefix – pertaining to the ear
otalgia	pain in the ear
otitis media	inflammation of the middle ear
otomy	suffix – a surgical incision performed for the removal of
otorrhoea	a discharge from the ear

ous	suffix – pertaining to
ox	prefix – pertaining to oxygen
oxia	suffix – oxygen, e.g. hypoxia
pachy	prefix – thick, e.g. pachydermo (thick/ elephant skin) periostitis
paed	prefix – pertaining to the child
Paget's disease	chronic bone disease to create softening and deformity. Progresses through a lytic, sclerotic, resting and possible sarcomatous phase
pan	prefix – total or all, e.g. pandemic
pancreatitis	inflammation of the pancreas
papill	prefix – protrusion/nipple, e.g. papilloma
papilloedema	optic disc swelling due to raised intracranial pressure
papilloma	a benign epithelial tissue tumour that grows outwards and has a vascular core
para	prefix – around, beside or beyond
paralytic ileus	obstruction of the intestine caused by loss of peristalsis. May also follow surgery or passing of gallstones
paraplegia	paralysis of both lower limbs
paresis	suffix – slight paralysis
Parkinson's disease	a degenerative brain disease linked to tremors or rigidity. Shaking of limbs may be termed Parkinsonism
path	prefix – disease
pathy	suffix – disease
penia	suffix – reduction in number or amount of, e.g. osteopenia
pepsia	suffix – pertaining to the digestion
per	prefix – through
peria	prefix – surrounding, outside, e.g. periosteum
pericardial effusion	an effusion (fluid collection) between the two layers of the pericardium
pericarditis	inflammation of the pericardium
peritonitis	inflammation of the peritoneum

Perthe's disease (Perthe–Legg–Calve disease)	aseptic necrosis of the epiphysis of the femoral head resulting in shape change to the articular surface
petit mal	epilepsy without the classical fitting episodes noted for grand mal epilepsy
petr	prefix – stone, e.g. osteopetrosis
pexy	suffix – surgical fixation, e.g. pneumopexy
phag	prefix – eat, swallow
phagia	suffix – eat, swallow
philia	suffix – love (attracted to), e.g. hydrophilic
phleb	prefix – pertaining to the veins
phlebitis	inflammation of a vein
phlebolith	a calcified thrombus in a vein. Radiographic differentiation shows a reduced density to the centre of the calcified region
phobia	suffix – aversion or abnormal fear of something
phonia	suffix – sound or voice
phoria	suffix – feeling, e.g. euphoria
phot	prefix – pertaining to light
physi	prefix – nature of, e.g. physiology
physis	suffix – growth, e.g. physis of a bone
placenta praevia	placenta in an abnormal position
plasia	suffix – growth, development or formation, e.g. neoplasis
plasm	suffix – growth, development or formation
plasty	suffix – surgical repair, e.g. arthroplasty
plegia	suffix – paralysis
pleural effusion	fluid between the two layers of the pleura
pleurisy	inflammation of the pleura – a dryness that creates pain as a lack of serous fluid causes rubbing of the layers on ventilation

pnea (pnoea)	suffix – breathing
pneum	prefix – pertaining to the lung (air or gas)
pneumoconiosis	lung disease resulting from dust particle inhalation
pneumonectomy	surgical removal of the lung
pneumoperitoneum	air or gas in the peritoneum, best revealed with an erect CXR
pneumothorax	presence of air in the pleural cavity to cause collapse of the lung
pod	prefix – pertaining to the foot
poiesis	suffix – formation of, e.g. haematopoiesis
poikil	prefix – irregular, varied, e.g. osteopoikilosis
poli	prefix – pertaining to the nervous grey matter
poliomyelitis	polio virus infection and inflammation of the spinal cord grey matter to cause loss of function
poly	prefix – many, multiple
polycythaemia	increased number of red blood cells in the blood supply
polydactyly	congenital presence of extra digits of the hand or foot
polyp	a protruberance of tissue of a stalk, termed sessile or pedunculate respectively, as the stalk lengthens in dimensions
polyuria	excess urine production
post	prefix – after
porosis	suffix – porosity, e.g. osteporosis
Pott's fracture	fracture of the lower end of tibia and fibula
pre	prefix – before
prim	prefix – first, e.g. primary
primigravida	a woman pregnant for the first time
primipara	a woman who has given birth to her first child
pro	prefix – before
proct	prefix – pertaining to the rectum

prolapse	abnormal descent or extrusion of a structure within or into a cavity
prostat	prefix – pertaining to the prostate gland
prostatectomy	surgical removal of the prostate gland
proximal	nearest to the centre or midline
pseud	prefix – false, e.g. pseudarthrosis
psoriasis	common skin disease with reddened scaly patches and a link to arthritic changes
psych	prefix – pertaining to the mind
ptosis	suffix – protruding, sagging, prolapse
ptysis	suffix – spitting, e.g. haemoptysis
puerper	prefix – childbirth
pulmon	prefix – pertaining to the lung
py(o)	prefix – relating to pus
pyel	prefix – relating to the renal pelvis
pyelonephritis	inflammation of the pelvis, calyces and nephrons of the kidney
pyloric stenosis	a narrowing of the pyloric canal with pathognomic projectile vomiting in the newborn, more frequent in males
pyr	prefix – heat
pyrexia	a raised temperature with associated fever
quadr	prefix – four
quadriplegia	paralysis of all limbs
radic	prefix – pertaining to the nerve root, e.g. radiculopathy
rect	prefix – pertaining to the rectum
renal	kidney
retin	prefix – pertaining to the retina of the eye
retro	prefix – behind or back
rhabd	prefix – rod-shaped, striated
rheumatic fever	an infection that may affect joints and valves of the heart

rheumatoid arthritis	chronic arthritis that affects a number of joints, most frequently the small joints. Appearances include periarticular erosions, joint space increase from swelling, then reduced joint space, loss of alignment of joints and osteoporotic change each side of the joint
rhin	prefix – pertaining to the nose
rhinorrhoea	fluid discharge from the nose
rrhagia	suffix – excessive flow, e.g. haemorrhage
rrhoea	suffix – discharge
rickets	softening bone deformity in childhood from vitamin D deficiency – cupping of epiphyses may also be noted
rugae	coarse folding of the mucosa of the stomach
salp	prefix – pertaining to the fallopian tubes
salpingitis	inflammation of the fallopian tubes
salpinx	suffix – fallopian tube
sarc	prefix – connective tissue
sarcoidosis	chronic inflammatory disease of unknown cause. Linked to arthritic changes and calcifications in the ear pinna and tip of the nose
sarcoma	suffix –malignant connective-tissue tumour, e.g. osteogenic sarcoma
Scheurmann's disease	aseptic necrosis of the vertebral bodies in younger adults, creates invaginations of the end plates termed Schmorl's nodes
sciatica	pain along the sciatic nerve from buttock to toes
sclerosis	suffix – hardening, stiffening, e.g. arteriosclerosis
scoli	prefix – curved, crooked

Appendix 2

scoliosis	lateral curvature of the spine – excessive in young adults would result in surgical intervention – may be evident with abdominal pain with convexity towards source of pain
scope	suffix – to look at, instrument for looking at, e.g. endoscope
scopy	suffix – visual examination, e.g. endoscopy
semi	prefix – half
seminoma	a tumour of the germinal epithelium of the seminiferous tubules of the testis
sepsis	suffix – infection
shingles	a viral infection (similar to chickenpox) of the adult nervous system
sial	prefix – pertaining to saliva
sinusitis	inflammation of the nasal sinuses
sis	suffix – state of
somat	prefix – body
somn	prefix – sleep
Spalding's sign	overlapping of skull bones to indicate foetal death
spasm	suffix – sudden involuntary contraction of muscle, e.g. vasospasm
sperm (spermat)	prefix – pertaining to sperm
sphygm	prefix – pulse, e.g. sphygmomanometer
spina bifida	congenital failure to fuse of the posterior neural arch of the vertebra
spir	prefix – breathe, e.g. spirometry
spleen	prefix – pertaining to the spleen
splenomegaly	enlargement of the spleen
spondyl	prefix – pertaining to vertebrae or the spinal column
spondylolisthesis	forward slipping of an upper vertebra on a lower vertebra due to spondylolysis or fracture of the pars interarticularis
spondylolysis	acute or chronic breakdown of the pars inter articularis
spondylosis	osteoarthritis of the spine

stalsis	suffix – contraction, e.g. peristalsis
staphyl	prefix – grape-like clusters, e.g. staphylococcus
stasis	suffix – control or stop, e.g. haemostasis
stenosis	narrowing of a previously patent passageway, e.g. mitral stenosis is a narrowing of the mitral valve between the left atrium and ventricle
steth	prefix – pertaining to the chest
Still's disease	juvenile rheumatoid arthritis
strept	prefix – twisted chains or links, e.g. streptococcus
stricture	narrowing of a passage
sub	prefix – under or lower
super	prefix – above or higher
supra	prefix – above
sym	prefix – joined or together
syn	prefix – joined or together
syndrome	a group of signs and symptoms of a disease
synovi	prefix – pertaining to the synovium
tachy	prefix – fast or rapid
tachycardia	abnormally rapid beating of the heart
ten(d)	prefix – tendon
tendin	prefix – tendon
tenosynovitis	inflammation of a tendon sheath
teratoma	a tumour of an organ or tissue that contains normal variations of all three germ layers; see dermoid cyst
test	prefix – pertaining to the testicles or testes
tetra	prefix – four
tetraplegia	paralysis of all limbs
thorax	suffix – pertaining to the chest
thoracoplasty	local collapse of a lung achieved by surgical removal of several ribs
thoracotomy	surgical opening into the thoracic cavity
thrombosis	clot formation within a blood vessel

Appendix 2

thromb	prefix – a clot of blood
thrombus	a blood clot
thym	prefix – pertaining to the thymus gland, e.g. thymoma
thyr	prefix – pertaining to the thyroid gland
thyrotoxicosis	overactivity of the thyroid gland
tinnitus	ringing (or high-pitched noise) in the ears
tom	prefix – to cut or section, e.g. tomography
tome	suffix – an instrument used to cut, e.g. osteotome
torticollis	twisting of the neck to turn the head towards the side associated with spasm of the neck muscles
tox	suffix – poison
toxic	prefix – poison
trache	prefix – pertaining to the trachea
trans	prefix – across, through or beyond
tri	prefix – three
trich	prefix – pertaining to the hair
tripsy	suffix – crushing surgically, e.g. lithotripsy
trophy	suffix – nourishment, growth, e.g. cytotrophy
tympan	prefix – middle ear, ear drum
ulcer	an open skin or membrane sore
ultra	prefix – beyond or extra
ungu	prefix – nail
uni	prefix – one
ur	prefix – pertaining to the urinary system
uraemia	symptoms associated with toxic substances in the bloodstream when the kidney fails to filter the material
uresis	suffix – micturition
uria	suffix – pertaining to urine or urination
uter	prefix – pertaining to the uterus
uvul	prefix – pertaining to the uvula

vagin	pertaining to a vagina, e.g. tenovaginitis where vagina means sheath, in this case for a tendon to pass through
Valsalva manoevre	forced expiration against a closed glottis to bring about a raised intrathoracic pressure
valv	prefix – pertaining to a valve
valvul	prefix – pertaining to a valve
varices	dilated veins
vas	prefix – vessel or duct, e.g. vas deferens
ven	prefix – pertaining to veins
ventricul	prefix – pertaining to the ventricles
vertebr	prefix – pertaining to the vertebrae or spinal column
vertigo	dizziness
vesic	prefix – pertaining to a bladder or sac
vesical calculus	a stone (calculus) in the urinary bladder
vesicul	prefix – pertaining to the seminal vesicles
viscer	prefix – pertaining to the internal organs
volvulus	a twisting of the bowel (caecum or sigmoid colon) to cause an obstruction
vulv	prefix – pertaining to the vulva
Wegener's granuloma	a highly malignant, destructive lesion of the nasopharynx
whiplash injury	acute, traumatic flexion extension injury of the cervical spine
Wilms' tumour	malignant kidney tumour, usually affecting young children
xanth	prefix – yellow
xer	prefix – dry
xerosis	dryness, most frequently of the skin

Appendix 3

Typical Normal Blood Values

Cellular make-up

Erythrocytes (red blood cells; RBC)	♂	$5.4 \times 10^6/\mu L$
	♀	$4.8 \times 10^6/\mu L$
Leukocytes (white blood cells; WBC)		$5-10 \times 10^3/\mu L$
	Neutrophils	60–70% of WBCs
	Eosinophils	2–4% of WBCs
	Basophils	0.5–1% of WBCs
	Lymphocytes	20–25% of WBCs
	Monocytes	3–8% of WBCs
Platelets		$150-400 \times 10^3/\mu L$

Index of Medical Imaging, First Edition. Jonathan McConnell.
© 2011 Blackwell Publishing Ltd. Published 2011 by Blackwell Publishing Ltd.

Measured values used to indicate disease

Bleeding time	<9.5 minutes, range 2–9 minutes
Prothrombin time (PT)	12–15 seconds
Haematocrit (% RBCs in blood)	♂ 40–54%, average 47% ♀ 38–46%, average 42%
Erythrocyte sedimentation rate (ESR) – increases with age	♂ <50 years <15 mm/h ♂ >50 years <20 mm/h ♀ <50 years <20 mm/h ♀ >50 years under 30 mm/h
Clotting/coagulation time	Range 2–8 minutes
Creatinine levels	♂ 0.6–1.2 mg/dL ♀ 0.5–1.1 mg/dL
Blood glucose levels	4–8 mmol/L normal range 3.5–7 mmol/L fasting Under 10 mmol/L after meals
Prostate-specific antigen	>3.9 ng/mL may indicate inflammation, infection or cancer